one heart, four seasons

Kundalini Yoga, Experience Present Moment Awareness

by Susan Quaglia Brown | *Sat Dharam Kaur*

illustrations by

Allison Cekala | *Ong Kar Kaur*

Published by
YOGA ART AWARENESS
251 Cram Hill Road
Lyndeborough, NH 03082
www.oneheartfourseasons.com

Copyright ©2010 by Susan Quaglia Brown
All rights reserved.

Illustrations by Allison Cekala
Book design by Teri Jankowski

PRINTED IN THE UNITED STATES OF AMERICA

Library of Congress Control Number: 2010916188
ISBN 978-0-615-40306-9

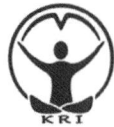

KRI Seal Statement: This publication has received the KRI Seal of Approval.
This Seal is given only to products that have been reviewed for accuracy and integrity
of the sections containing the 3HO lifestyle and Kundalini Yoga as taught by Yogi Bhajan®.

All teachings, yoga sets, techniques, kriyas and meditations
courtesy of The Teachings of Yogi Bhajan. Reprinted with permission.
Unauthorized duplication is a violation of applicable laws. ALL RIGHTS RESERVED.
No part of these Teachings may be reproduced or transmitted in any form
by any means, electronic or mechanical, including photocopying and recording,
or by any information storage and retrieval system, except as may be
expressly permitted in writing by The Teachings of Yogi Bhajan.

To request permission, please write to
KRI at PO Box 1819, Santa Cruz, NM 87567 or see www.kriteachings.org

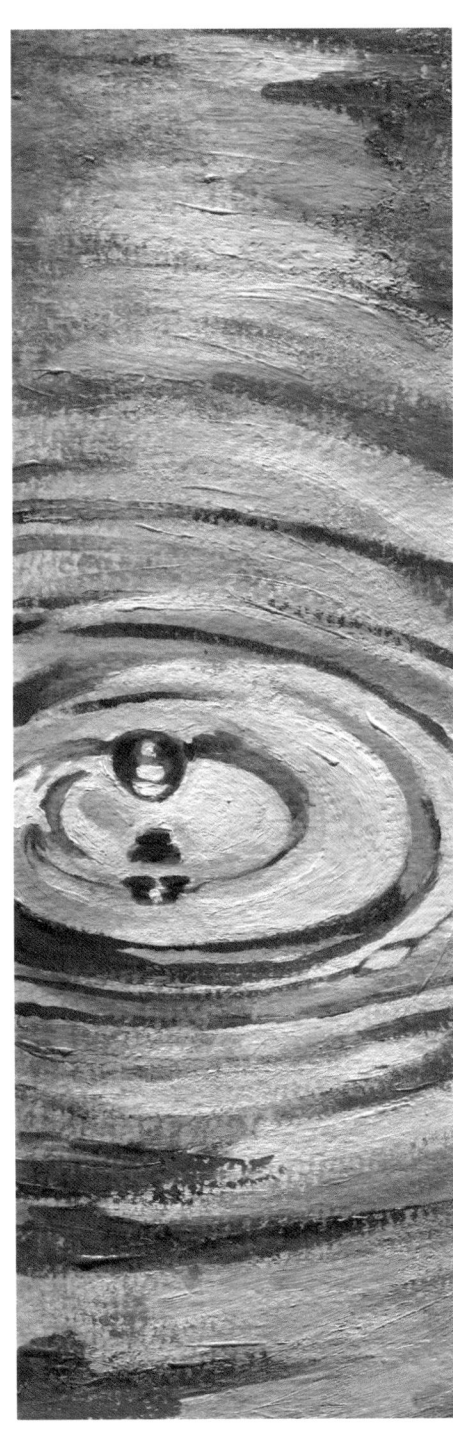

this book is dedicated to

my two beautiful sons,
Sean and Evan;

to Allison,
who is like a daughter to me;

and to my beloved husband,
Aaron;

with love.

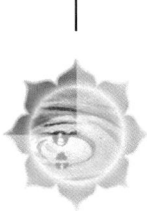

acknowledgements

Immeasurable depths of gratitude and love to Yogi Bhajan,
for bringing Kundalini Yoga to the West.

blessings to

Gurucharan Singh Khalsa, PhD,
for your tireless service bringing Yogi Bhajan's teachings to all;

Hari Kirin Kaur Khalsa,
for bringing friendship and Kundalini Yoga to me;

L. Lyedecker Geer,
my friend of 25 years
for traveling with me every step of the way;

And to Siri Neel Kaur Khalsa
for your graceful support and wisdom too great to measure.

Wahe Guru!

thank you

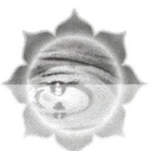

Enid Ames, Libby Barnett, Laurie Boyle, Aaron Brown, Emmaline Brown, Erik Brown, Laura Bullock, Allison Cekala, Lauren Chorazak, Evan Coronis, Samuel Coronis, Sean Coronis, Hrdayasakti/Christine Eaton, Sarah Buck Garcia, Lyedie Geer, Carol Thompson Hess, Kristina Klee-Horning, Helaine Iris, Teri Jankowski, Larry Kennedy, Patty Quaglia Kennedy, Bakshish Kaur Khalsa, Hari Kirin Kaur Khalsa, Zoe Lantaff, Dana Marangi/Nirankar Kaur, Gary Pinette, Patrice Pinette, Dorothy Quaglia, Frank M. Quaglia I, Lucille Quaglia, Michael Quaglia, Carol Renwick, Diego Sharon, Randi Stein, Susan Prince Thompson, Anne Quaglia Trane, David Trane, Diane Trane, Romulo Valdez Jr., Ph.D, Melissa White, Jery Whitworth, Kristina Wilson and Blake Wood for believing in me. Sat Nam.

*Thank you to models for posing for the drawings:
Aaron T. Brown, Emmaline Brown, Susan Q. Brown, Andrew Cekala, Allison Cekala, Ben Cloutier, Evan Coronis, Sean Coronis, Graceon Cyr, Lea Cyr, Lindsay Dozoretz, Shirin Khosravi, Jill McCullough, Nick Miller, Mackenzie Moore, Suzanne Moore, Narisa Richard and Sarah Skenazy.*

*Allison and I had a lot of fun deciding on how to make the instructional drawings for this book. We wanted to use many different ages and body types. So while we are striving for perfection in the poses, **reality** also shines through! Strive for perfection in your poses and love the reality that you are!*

a special thank you

To the three women who supported me in this project:
Teri Jankowski, Laura Bullock and Allison Cekala.

I met Allison Cekala three years ago at Kripalu in Lenox, MA where I was teaching a Kundalini Yoga set for sadhana. We are doing Yoga together still, and she is a friend and daughter to me for time eternal. Allison is a gifted artist, musician and Yoga teacher. She made all of the beautiful drawings for this book, and her graceful presence has infused the artwork with joy and prana.

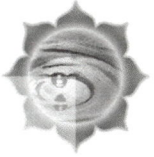

Teri Jankowski was a gift from the saints and angels, and she walked into my life and changed it forever with her excitement to design the cover and layout for this book. Teri is an international book design award winner; a tireless vital participant in her brother's organization, citta.org; a wise woman healer; a partner in her husband's business, Don Thomas Music; and a dear sister-friend to me.

Laura Bullock, referred to me by Teri, has been a clear editing voice and stable presence from the first e-mail communication to the last. I so appreciate her patience with me as a first-time author! I've enjoyed her intelligence, warmth and joyful honesty during our collaboration. She flowed patiently with the Divine Grace that sustains us all.

All Kundalini Yoga kriyas and meditations in this book were taught by Yogi Bhajan between 1968 until his death in 2004. Whenever I say *Kundalini Yoga*, I am referring to Kundalini Yoga as taught by Yogi Bhajan®.

Using a particular practice for each season is my concept for this book and is not a practice that Yogi Bhajan taught.

Always consult your doctor before beginning this or any other exercise program. Nothing in this book is to be construed as medical advice. The benefits attributed to the practice of Kundalini Yoga come from the centuries old Yogic traditions. Results will vary with individuals.

Do not practice Kundalini Yoga under the influence of recreational drugs.

If you have any questions or concerns, please consult me at www.oneheartfourseasons.com.

May I be forgiven for any mistakes or omissions.
Sat Nam.

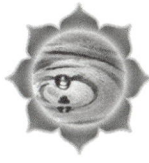

contents

iii . . . . *foreword*
v . . . . *preface*
ix . . . . *introduction*
xix . . . . *using this book*

1 . . . . solstice and equinox
3 . . . . my practice
5 . . . . when to practice
7 . . . . getting started
9 . . . . yoga kriyas
11 . . . . practicing
15 . . . . body locks to seal energy
19 . . . . breath (pranayam)
21 . . . . practicing pranayam
27 . . . . mantra
29 . . . . mudra / hand positions
31 . . . . focal point for your eyes
33 . . . . meditation
35 . . . . how to sit, stand and bend
45 . . . . energy centers in the body
53 . . . . tune in to begin
57 . . . . practice for present moment awareness

contents (continued)

59 . . . . to end
61 . . . . always
63 . . . . warm-ups
81 . . . . a meditation and kriya for all seasons
85 . . . . *spring equinox*
93 . . . . *midsummer solstice*
103 . . . . *autumn equinox*
111 . . . . *midwinter solstice*
121 . . . . tantric meditation
125 . . . . journaling after yoga

131 . . . . *source glossary*
133 . . . . *glossary of gurmuki and sanskrit terms*
137 . . . . *bibliography*
139 . . . . *references*

144 . . . . *notes*

foreword by Jery Whitworth

In **One Heart, Four Seasons**, Susan Quaglia Brown draws from her 25 years of in-depth Yoga and meditation practice to demystify Kundalini Yoga. Out from under its previous misleading portrayal, Susan skillfully reframes Kundalini Yoga as a valuable tool to assist individuals through difficult situations and challenges one faces. Assisting the physical body to surrender and release its blockages and pain, Yoga aids in fighting fatigue, helps to overcome and transition through illnesses, increases flexibility and strength, and enhances the immune system.

Susan's Kundalini Yoga teaching approach uniquely sets itself apart from others. Ms. Brown is keenly aware of varied differences in body types and levels of expertise in those exploring her method. Her flexible coaching style 'strives for perfection while meeting you where you are at' on your own individual journey. Providing many variations towards an optimal pose, Susan's wide range of options lead the reader not only towards ways to incorporate this practice into daily life, but also how to derive a wide range of mind, body, spirit, and energetic benefits.

In Susan's approach, yoga sets and meditations are coordinated with the Four Seasons to synchronize one's body and mind with the cycles and vibrational energy of Nature resulting in a deepening of the process. In this heightened state of focused awareness, where quieting of the "monkey" mind" chatter occurs, the participant/reader is transported on a safe and gentle journey of self-exploration which soothe and liberate emotional stressors and tensions.

Whether you are new to Kundalini Yoga, or a seasoned veteran of its practice, a high degree of consideration and attention to all levels of experience is present in Ms. Brown's teaching. Her unique instructional approach reshapes "standards or goals of perception that are exclusive" into an approachable and tangible practice for all walks of life, body types, and ages.

Within Susan's insightful and mindful book awaits numerous rewarding possibilities. There could be no better time than now to EXPERIENCE the experience of Susan Brown's Kundalini Yoga heart-felt teachings.

preface

I was born three weeks premature and spent my first week on earth in an incubator, warm, attended to and separated from my mother. She cried from her hospital bed, wanting us to be snuggled-in together. Years later, as an adult, I believed that my birth was mismanaged and therefore caused unnecessary suffering. It was after the birth of my first child, during meditation, that I remembered my experience in the incubator: bright fluorescent lights and the whirring sounds of motion-filled life softened by the glass enclosure of my mechanical cocoon; I remembered it!

I was not alone. A presence, beautiful beyond description, was with me. I did not feel alone at all and I had no thoughts or judgments. There was no sense of time. I was part of a loving presence, and that is all there was. Experiencing an eternity of pure love was how I began this life. I forgot all of this, descending into the spell of matter, experiencing its relentless duality: pleasure and pain, good and bad, like and dislike.

As a child and into young adulthood, I spent long hours outside in the woods and fields surrounding our house in Massachusetts. I was hungry for magical stories: I was seeking *something*. Eventually, after doing Hatha Yoga and meditating for more than a decade, I met my dear friend, Joan Hanley, also known as Hari Kirin Kaur. We practiced *her* Yoga, Kundalini Yoga, for nearly every day together for a year. Hari Kirin Kaur learned from Yogi Bhajan directly, and as she shared these teachings with me, I knew that I was receiving an auspicious gift. Practicing Kundalini Yoga as taught by Yogi Bhajan®, I learned to sustain present moment awareness and peace in the midst of a complex divorce. I began to seriously investigate this incredible Yoga.

Yogi Bhajan[1] (1929-2004) was born in British India in the province of Punjab. He was a Master of Kundalini Yoga (for which he is best known) by age 16. Kundalini Yoga is Raj Yoga, the mother of all Yoga, the Yoga of awareness practiced by the householder, which typifies Yogi Bhajan's teachings: living your true identity, as Finite Self and Infinite Self united, while fully engaged in the world. This is another way of saying *living in present moment awareness*. The Gurmukhi mantra *Sat Nam* means *true name*. *Sat* can also be translated to mean the *infinite* or *heaven*, and *Nam* can be translated to mean *earth* or the *manifested world*. Your true identity creates heaven on earth, now.

Yogi Bhajan gave me my spiritual name, Sat Dharam Kaur, which means *Princess of the True Path*.

I flowed with the grace and practice, becoming a certified Level I teacher, and for several years taught Kundalini Yoga as taught by Yogi Bhajan® to adults and teens. Then, for three years (2006-08), I helped create and co-owned the Kundalini Yoga Studio & Art Gallery with Hari Kirin Kaur Khalsa in New Hampshire. We're the artists in town who practice Yoga, and we have worked together for more than a decade to integrate art and Yoga as material for site-specific public art installations. I now teach Kundalini Yoga and make art from my studio Yoga Art Awareness (YAA) in Lyndeborough, New Hampshire.

Three decades of art, including paintings, works on paper and public art, reflect my career-long meditation on the reconciliation between heaven and earth. Making art brings me to stillness. Painting, combined with Yoga, meditation and singing and chanting have been my spiritual practice for more than 25 years. Studio as sanctuary has produced many miracles, and the peace of present moment awareness lives in the paintings. Singing, meditation and chanting are part of the paint.

As the manuscript for this book was being completed, I was talking to my Tuesday morning class about Yoga, life and my book and a student suggested that I title it *Becoming Normal*. We all laughed because we deeply understood the truth of her words. If you are new to Yoga, you may have ideas about Yoga that some Westerners share, such as: You need to be flexible to do Yoga. Yoga is mysterious or weird. Yoga is too easy. It is only for girls. Or, you can't be Catholic, Protestant, Christian, Muslim, or Jewish and do Yoga.

Yoga is not a religion. Yoga uses normal everyday processes that happen to everybody every day; breathing, moving and vocalizing. In Yoga, you consciously direct your breathing, moving and vocalizing to *normalize* your awareness. Normal by definition means: usual, healthy and occurring naturally. Your normal awareness, which is healthy and occurring naturally, is unchanging stillness and peace! Kundalini Yoga delivers you to your normal awareness or true identity! Eventually it becomes common to know that this peace is who you are! You must experience it to believe the simple and powerful elegance of Yoga technology.

To Yogi Bhajan, I feel the deepest appreciation, love and gratitude. Thank you! I am so happy that you brought this ancient then-secret technology to America in 1968 for everyone to experience. Practicing this Yoga and meditation has served me well and your guidance resides in my heart and dreams. I have evolved from an infant experiencing the grace of radiant presence to an adult consciously living life *as* radiant presence, living as an eternity of pure love. Now. Wahe Guru!

Wahe Guru means …*Indescribable is the ecstasy of the wisdom, the grace that brings us from darkness to light.*

introduction

Why is this book different from other Yoga books? It makes available tools to deepen and sustain your experience of the Now. This book will help you to design a Kundalini Yoga practice that follows the natural rhythms of the earth's rotation cycles around the sun. Practicing Yoga is about learning to follow your own rhythms, responding to what is real in your life and discovering that all the while, inner stillness is present. Learning how to notice stillness is a powerful practice. Stillness can only be experienced now.

Experiencing the Now is liberation from suffering. Using this book will teach you how to be present to the totality of you: body, mind and spirit, while cognitive and connecting to the world in which we live. You will learn how to strengthen your physical body. You will learn how to open through your Divine Heart and release unconscious fears, angers and limiting beliefs. You will learn to replace egoic suffering with the clarity of present moment awareness. Eckhart Tolle, in his book, *A New Earth,* has guided millions of people to investigate the Now. This book gives you tools to experience the Now.

You will feel peace, reduce stress and become fit, living in the West using Yoga originating from the East. Yoga, when artfully practiced, is a powerful technology for health. Kundalini Yoga is more than 5,000 years old. It's a proven technology and it works for all ages and abilities. Even if you only have 15 minutes each day to spend, you will find short exercises and meditations in this book that will work for you. If you have more time, the real difference and profound benefit of Kundalini Yoga as taught by Yogi Bhajan® is the practice of kriya — a complete set of exercises — a completed action.

Kundalini Yoga, practiced as directed, is a precise technology that will produce noticeable results immediately. A calm mind, peaceful heart and beautiful body will develop with regular practice called *sadhana*. Kundalini Yoga integrates body, mind and spirit in your personal relationships and at work, in the world and at home. It is an ancient technology, time-tested and effective.

Yogi Bhajan said, "Try your best and let the universe do the rest." *Try your best* is your opportunity to practice Kundalini Yoga and *Let the universe do the rest* is the responding Grace. It always responds.

Kundalini Yoga as taught by Yogi Bhajan® uses prescribed postures, breath techniques, mantras and meditations. It is also a moment-to-moment sadhana devoted to integrating your finite, egoic self with your infinite, Divine Self. This delivers you to the present moment. You do this by opening through your heart and trusting the Divine Will to do the rest.

Kundalini Yoga is a practice that uses traditional Yoga technology. This is why I am so excited about sharing Kundalini Yoga with you. The practice of relating through your open heart, where all stress dissolves, is the key. All good things flow from there. Your open heart is stress-free and knows when to move and do postures and meditations and when to be outwardly still, not using postures or meditations.

Kundalini Yoga practice is not done to become more flexible, although that will happen.
Kundalini Yoga practice is not about recognizing enlightenment, although that may happen.
Kundalini Yoga practice is about seeing the Divine in all things and living according to Divine Will, of which you are a part. Opening and surrendering through the heart is the practice of experiencing the present moment, always part of the creative and sustaining force in the universe, always Now.

My meditation practice has taught me that spiritual reality includes all that you can see, feel, touch, and experience, as well as freedom from what you can see, feel, touch, and experience. Welcome to East meets West. This means that you experience liberation of Infinite Consciousness, also called the un-manifested and the entirety of the manifest world.

In ordinary terms, *liberation of Infinite Consciousness and the entirety of the manifest world* means that you are totally relaxed and free from all stress and worry to such an extent that you feel love for everything. You are in a state of grace that is totally human. Enlightenment is experienced by fully opening through the heart to both emptiness and fullness. Both are parts of a whole and inseparable, like the in-breath and out-breath that sustain your life.

This is so hard to explain because *liberation of Infinite Consciousness* is formless and without content, that's why it is so wonderful and still and *Awake*. The following is my personal story to help explain *emptiness*.

I love to keep a dream journal and have done so for more than a decade. I have experienced lucid dreaming, dreaming when you remain conscious that you are dreaming while asleep, on many occasions. Having read that Sri Ramana Maharshi and Sri Aurobundo and Ken Wilber all remained conscious in formless dreamless sleep, I decided that I would like to experience this, too!

Finding myself at a hypnotherapy session with a family member to help them quit smoking, I asked the therapist, who is a friend of mine, if we could insert two more suggestions at the end of the session. My first intention was to quit snoring (why not?) and the second was to remain conscious during formless dreamless sleep. Maharshi taught that what remains in formless dreamless sleep is the true self.

The family member did quit smoking, and several months after the session, still snoring, something funny and profound happened to me. One night while I was in bed sleeping, my husband lightly elbowed me and said, "You are snoring!"

But before he said that, and before I woke up, for a brief eternal moment, I was conscious in formless dreamless sleep! It seemed to last forever and was so ordinary in its extraordinariness! Eckhart Tolle calls it stillness, and I understand why, because it is still and without content or form, but I call it *Awakeness*! My awareness was so AWAKE in formlessness! Amazing. And all the while I was snoring like a freight train!

Those few moments of awake awareness or stillness continue to inform my life. That awareness or the *unmanifested* is always available to me, even now as I write I can feel the awake aware presence that is all of life, that is me. It is aware through my eyes and it has no eyes!

And the doing part, the *manifested* — the arising and falling of everyone talking, eating, sleeping, moving, breathing, snoring, loving, hating, playing, working, living, dying, behaving, misbehaving, giving, taking — all of it is experienced by me as one thing. I cannot forget because I experienced that every possible reality is happening in the universe every moment and it is one "doing." Each moment, aka Now, only one thing is happening! It just happens to be all of creation! "One is doing," Ken Wilber said, "something is doing, we don't know what." That's for sure!

The really funny part is that we all are already enlightened right now. Every one is. It's impossible not to be. Right now, you are awake and aware beyond all thoughts and feelings: What remains, during formless, dreamless sleep is constant, it is reality. It's just that you are distracted by your thoughts, and you have not been taught how to notice the stillness of the present moment and sustain that awareness. If you have ever experienced, while driving a car, that for a few seconds or longer you were so lost in thought that you forgot that you were driving, this is what I am talking about. Your own observation that you were not paying attention alerted you to reality. If you did not notice, an accident would've likely resulted.

Ideas like this illustrate that you can be separate from any aspect of life and those ideas are sometimes really loud. In the example I gave in the previous paragraph, of driving the car, you were still really driving, regardless of your thoughts, which caused you to momentarily *forget* that you were driving a car! Thoughts can drown out the stillness that *drives* your life and is always present. The concepts you believe prevent you from realizing this pervasive stillness. In any given moment, the story in your head, especially if you have forgotten that you are thinking, determines your focus and experience. Noticing that you are thinking can begin the process of bringing your feet down to earth and out of the clouds of mental fantasy.

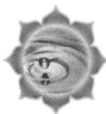

Once you begin to practice Kundalini Yoga, you begin the process of awakening and grounding to your true identity. With every breath, practicing Kundalini Yoga as directed, you may have a direct experience of the intention behind all Yogas since the first Yogic breath was realized: union. Yoga means *union*, specifically union between your egoic, finite self and your infinite self or in the words of Yogi Ramana Maharshi, *I-I. I am-ness* brings together spiritual awareness of the East with material attainment of the West.

The Yoga master, Sri Aurobindo (1872-1950), taught that this union is about creating a new heaven and a new earth, not from your egoic thinking mind but from surrendering through your own heart.

Surrendering to the indescribable, unnamable Supreme Heart that gives you each breath, each thought, each moment, is pure bliss. This experience makes you more loving, compassionate, powerful, and successful in your relationships and at work. This book will teach you not only how to do Kundalini Yoga as taught by Yogi Bhajan® but also how to practice Kundalini Yoga as true identity.

To start, it is as simple as noticing that your breath is happening. Everyone can do it. It is as simple as noticing that you are thinking, breathing, reading, doing. You have all that is required, right now, to begin. All you need is the you that notices what you are doing. This is your awareness that brings you to the present moment where you ask, "Who is noticing?" Try it right now and notice who is noticing that you are reading these words.

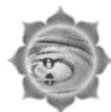

Do you want to respond to the awakening consciousness of our present day where intuition informs your intellect and body and spirit are harmonized? If you do, then use this book and design a regular Yoga practice that works for you! Beginning right where you are and regularly practicing Kundalini Yoga may bring about a powerful transformation. It's safe and effective. Just do it as directed, just as it's been practiced for thousands of years. Practice to become what you already are: liberated and at peace knowing that happiness has arrived.

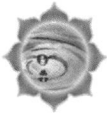

So what does all of that mean, and how do you use this book?

The expressions, *rising up and descending down,* refer to energy called Kundalini energy, which moves from the base of your spine up through energy centers (page 45) along your spine and then down again. When your own energy (Kundalini) rises up to the top of the spine and then descends down, it mixes in the middle at your heart center known as the heart chakra. This mixing and mingling of energy at the heart center allows wisdom, intuition and compassion to combine with passion, intellect and doing. You are normalizing your awareness.

When the Kundalini energy rises, it gives you tremendous energy. Practicing Yoga consciously directs this powerful energy, which is your own energy with which you were born, back down to the base of the spine. This is the beginning of Yogic union. Why? Because your human ego is then transformed, and it is now working to serve your life with compassion for yourself, your family, community, and all beings.

Love makes Kundalini rise. It is that organic! Just watch a loving mother with her child, and you observe this truth put into practice. By surrendering your practice to your Infinite Heart, also called the Divine Shakti, you will feel the bliss that is your birthright. Your open heart, in and of itself, frees the Kundalini energy to rise from the base of the spine and connect your egoic self, which is dealing with survival, creativity, passion, and power, with your highest wisdom of compassion, truth, intuition, and interconnectedness. The Kundalini energy then brings that higher consciousness back down, descending into daily life.

Kundalini Yoga will give you tools for a practice that will allow you to be aware of the stillness and peace that is always, always, always present 100% of the time. Kundalini will give you tools to be present in the moment for whatever is happening, changing and being created by you and around you. In my Yoga and meditation practice, I have come to understand that conscious integration of body, mind, soul, and spirit is the evolutionary stage that we are experiencing now at this time in the history of human consciousness.

Ken Wilber has outlined in his book, *Integral Spirituality,* that as wonderful as experiencing I-I is, it is still a form of arrogance without your devotion through your heart. If you do not open through your heart, your mind is closed and your witnessing presence, I-I, is not enough to humble your ego into emptiness. That is why Sri Aurobindo called surrendering through the heart to the Divine Shakti, Integral Yoga. Surrendering as devotion through your heart and witnessing as I-I allows your ego to dissolve into your true identity, Sat Nam. Welcome to integration of all aspects of your being. It is heaven on earth. Fragmentation ends. You are planting seeds for peace.

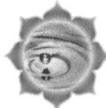

I have suggested chanting meditations for each season or section of this book. For centuries, these meditations have worked to powerfully open the heart and they will open your heart if practiced as directed.

Enlightenment or present moment awareness is always your true self, always present, always now, still, and unchanging within the moment-to-moment flow of life's sensations and events. I am so grateful to the following persons for sharing their stories and wisdom pointing to the path, always Now, to peace:

When Yogi Bhajan came to the United States in 1968 to teach Yoga, he witnessed the great need for a powerful remedy that would respond to the turbulent times. Yogi Bhajan fell in love with the flower children, the hippies, and saw their suffering; he understood that they were searching for spiritual truths and that drugs could not deliver the liberation they were seeking. Because practicing Kundalini Yoga delivers one to the neutral mind beyond duality, he decided to break the taboo of teaching Kundalini Yoga openly and in California taught these teachings to everyone. If you are not experiencing the neutral mind, your heart is closed 100% of the time.

Yogi Bhajan taught Kundalini Yoga in colleges, churches, private homes, and YMCA's and at numerous rock concerts in the U.S during the 1970s. Upon hearing *Longtime Sunshine,* he decided that the song should be sung at the end of every Kundalini Yoga class as a tribute to those beautiful souls, the flower children, who sacrificed so much while trying to break out of cultural patterns that perpetuate war, class systems and discrimination. Yogi Bhajan established the mother ashram or home for Kundalini Yoga in Espanola, New Mexico. For more information about Yogi Bhajan, visit the 3HO.org website and check out the bibliography at the back of this book.

Sri Aurobindo developed Integral Yoga, which uses self-surrender and allows Grace or Shakti, the Divine Feminine, to accomplish inner transformation from egoic suffering to enlightenment or Supermind, as sadhana or spiritual practice. Surrender must happen from the heart, seen by the ancients as a gateway to the Divine, and is in itself the form of meditation or prayer that defines Integral Yoga. No other techniques are necessary — not mantras, postures, controlled breathing, or prescribed meditations. The end of suffering is accomplished by surrendering the egoic personality to the Divine Mother or Shakti. This is a powerful sadhana and is practiced every day as often as possible. For more about Aurobindo and some of the books he has written, see the bibliography at the back of this book.

Sri Ramana Maharshi attained spontaneous enlightenment at the age of 16 and is considered to be one of the most significant teachers to emerge from India during the early to mid 1900s. Most of his teachings were given in complete silence from his mountain pilgrimage in Arunachala in South India. His spiritual presence was enough to quiet the minds of his students and they received his teaching from their deepest knowing in their own being as present moment awareness. In his later years, he would also speak his teachings to persons who could not receive them in silence.

Encompassing Sri Ramana Marharshi's teachings is the experience of your true essence, which he taught: *that which remains in formless dreamless sleep.* Ramana Maharshi's teachinngs are at the heart of Eckhart Tolle's teachings.

Tsultrim Allione is one of the first contemporary feminist Western women to be ordained a Tibetan Buddhist nun. Allione has developed teaching methods that facilitate the Western mind to understand Eastern Buddhist philosophy and practice. Her book, *Women of Wisdom,* offers insight into six great women who have achieved full illumination in their day and some cultural challenges particular to them and their time in history.

Eckhart Tolle , author of *The Power of Now* and *A New Earth: Awakening to Your Life's Purpose,* is an example of a human being living as enlightened consciousness, free from any prescribed spiritual tradition or dogma but rather living as a meditative existence that is not diminished by his dynamic work in the world. Tolle's writings use many examples, including spiritual traditions from the East and West, which illuminate his journey of living without suffering or identification with egoic thinking. *See bibliography.*

Ken Wilber is considered one of the greatest philosophers of our time. He has written many books about his Integral Map of Consciousness. Wilber's integral model, (four quadrants, levels, lines, states, and types) and his philosophy for Integral Life Practice are based on his own decades-long meditation practice as well as his research of many well-known scholars, spiritual masters, philosophers, educators, doctors of psychology, scientists, and most notably on the writings of Sri Aurobindo and Sri Ramana Maharshi. *See bibliography.*

Byron Katie is a remarkable example of a contemporary woman living in absolute freedom from suffering, 100% of the time. She doesn't use the word *enlightenment* but instead says that she woke up to reality after a severe depression. When her method, *The Work,* is applied, it ends egoic identification with thought and is simple, elegant and works! In the preface to her book, *A Thousand Names for Joy,* Katie also says, "I discovered that when I believed my thoughts, I suffered, but that when I didn't believe them, I didn't suffer, and that this is true for every human being. Freedom is as simple as that. I found suffering is optional. I found a joy within me that has never disappeared, not for a single moment. That joy is in everyone, always."

using this book

Throughout the text, you'll come across some traditional Sanskrit words, some of which will be familiar to you if you already practice Yoga. For those of you who are new to Kundalini Yoga, there are words in Sanskrit [1A] and Gurmukhi.[1B]

- *Sanskrit is a historical Indo-Aryan language, one of the liturgical languages of Hinduism and Buddhism, and one of the 22 official languages of India.*

- *Gurmukhi, a script created by Guru Angad Dev Ji (1504-1552), is a phonetic alphabet for pronouncing sacred songs of different linguistic origins that later became the basis for Old Punjabi.*

Both languages originated in India. I have included all of these words, listed alphabetically, in a glossary at the back of the book.

I also have included a bibliography of all the books that I have used for reference to write this book so that you can go more deeply into your understanding of how to cultivate a practice that truly integrates body, mind and spirit. Exercising the mind, like exercising the body, is exciting when you gain knowledge to nourish the spirit. I invite you to check out the bibliography at the back.

And . . .

There is no substitute for direct experience, so as you read, if you find some of the concepts in this book about Yoga and meditation new or confusing, don't be discouraged. You have all that you need to begin now. Simply follow the instructions and do some Yoga. Notice the concepts begin to make sense as you experience the power of Yoga for yourself.

Sat Nam[2] is a mantra used frequently in Kundalini Yoga. *Sat* means truth and *Nam* means *identity*. *True identity* means *no separation*. *True identity* means that you and the creative life force are one. *Sat* can also be interpreted to mean *being*.[3] So *Sat Nam* also means *being identity* or an *identity of being*.

In Yogic philosophy, G.O.D. means the Generating, Organizing and Delivering/Destroying Principle, the Formless Consciousness everywhere, always. Yogi Bhajan said, "If you can't see God in all, you can't see God at all."[3A]

So what does this have to do with Yoga?

Yoga means *union*. *Human being* means *light-mind now*. I have to repeat this! *Human being* means *light-mind now*.

> **hu** = light
> **man** = mental
> **being** = now

In other words, you are a spiritual being or primordial non-dual consciousness in a physical body having a human experience for joy. Always Now.

In this moment, the *you* that is aware that you are reading this book, holding this book, thinking about these concepts, is the *I* that is always aware of the *I* that is thinking, reading and doing. Yogi Ramana Maharshi called this I-I the infinite I or the witness that is aware of the egoic, personal I. The witness and the personal are one mind. If you forget about one half of your mind, life doesn't go very well for you. If you live only as witness, you are not able to function in the world. If you live only as your personal ego, your heart is closed and you create suffering for yourself and others. Practicing Yoga and meditation give you the experience of your true identity as witness to formless consciousness, as witness to your soul, as witness to your body, as witness to your mind, and as witness to your spirit as one mind, Now.

Sat Nam is the truth of what you are, and lacking awareness of it, you unconsciously identify with thoughts arising out of duality and illusion: pleasure/pain, flexible/inflexible, female/male, and on and on endlessly volleying between the polarities of thinking, believing that you are this or that and believing that you are not this or not that. In truth, you are not your thoughts, you are not your body and you are not your soul or the world around you. Of course you **have** thoughts, you **have** a body, you **have** a soul, and you are living in the world. However, your true identity, the witnessing presence, can never be destroyed. As a spiritual being living in a physical body, the totality of you is alive, free, engaging in life with passion, feeling, thinking, doing, and cultivating life as I-I. Yogis say, "Just this." Before each breath, before each mantra or posture, feel the truth of what you are. And ask yourself, "Who wants to know?"

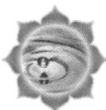

Breath awareness (pranayam), while doing the postures (asanas) and meditations, brings immediate noticeable results. Kundalini Yoga is a powerful technology that has only been available in the West since Yogi Bhajan brought it to us in 1968. Prior to that, it was taught in secret in India. Kundalini Yoga is here now, to help at a time when human consciousness is awakening to a new awareness as compassion and interconnectedness. Yogi Bhajan brought us this technology to help transition from the Piscean Age to the Aquarian Age. He explained that the Piscean Age was about *to be* or *not to be* and the Aquarian Age is about *to be, to be*.

About this transition to a new age Yogi Bhajan said,

> *The time has come of self-value. And the question is not 'To be or not to be.'*
> *The statement is 'To be, to be.' 'I am I am.' The time has come not to search for God, but to be God.*
> *Time is not to worship God, but to trust and dwell in the working of God.*[3B]

The Aquarian Age is Now. It can be found in the present moment.

Kundalini Yoga and meditation unite you to your compassionate heart, delivering you to the neutral mind, also called shuniya or present moment awareness. This state of being is the end of psychological suffering. Unhappy, angry, lonely, depressed, or afraid feelings are uncomfortable and hard to live with by design. They are your wake up call, and like an annoying alarm clock, they let you know that you have forgotten your true identity and are identifying with thinking. It is a reminder to access the I-I. It can't leave you and is always now present, is always now reality. Kundalini Yoga is a technology that, when used as directed, will bring you to an awakened awareness. This awareness is not something that is done to you; it is your own natural relaxed peaceful state, free from stress. You simply need to get quiet enough to see your own happy self. From that place of natural neutrality, you will peacefully create your life with joy.

This awakened awareness is not your thoughts and cannot be understood by thinking; thoughts are mental energy forms that allow you to create your world. You do not create your thoughts! They arise in response to your conscious or unconscious emotions, impartially, to give you your life. They are unbiased servants! When you dis-identify with your thoughts and remember that they are not you, and when you observe thoughts as a witnessing presence, you are free. You do this by noticing *who* is noticing *whom*, the I-I.

Experiencing this liberation that is always now present ends feelings of separation and identification with illusion. If you are not experiencing neutrality, the ego may tell you that liberation from thinking is boring. The ego from duality may tell you that the enlightened mind just sits around all day, too holy for doing or having fun. The truth is that the neutral mind or present moment awareness is a return to reality and allows you to have a human experience with joy. Active, juicy, feeling awake, fully participating in life!

The neutral mind is awakened awareness, stillness and peace on and off the Yoga mat. Experiencing your life from the neutral mind allows the gifts of reality to flow through you as joy: flexible or not, happy or sad, as a man or a woman. I-I. There is no greater peace activism than experiencing neutrality. Sat Nam.

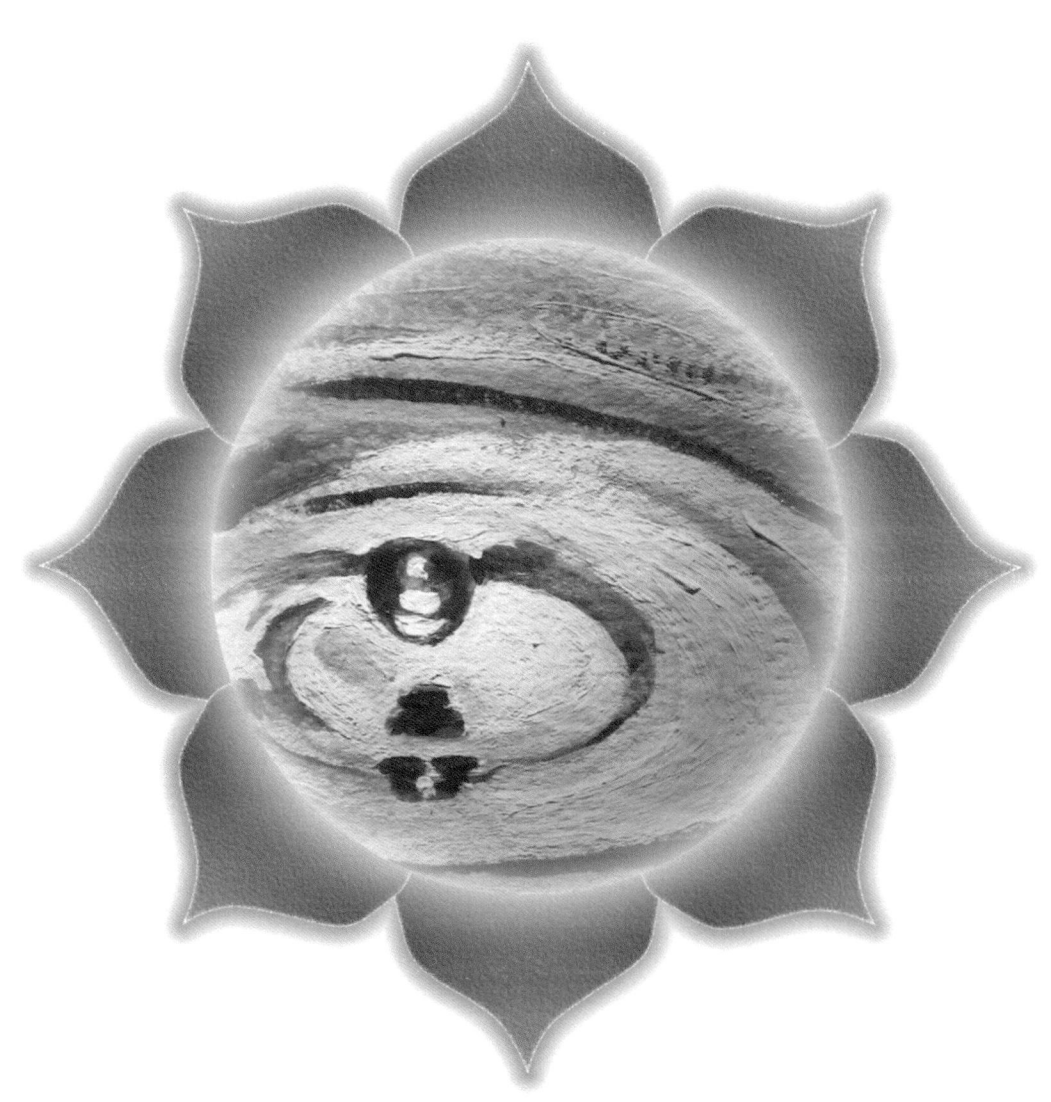

one heart, four seasons

Kundalini Yoga, Experience Present Moment Awareness

solstice and equinox

Revolve your life around Summer and Winter Solstice and everything will be taken care of.

— Yogi Bhajan[3c]

At approximately the 21st day of every third month of a calendar year, we have a solstice, *sol sistere*, which means *sun to stand still* or an equinox, *aequus nox*, which means *equal night*. The solstice occurs in summer and winter when the tilt of the earth's axis is directly towards or away from the sun.

Solstice

Northern Hemisphere

In June, the summer sun is directly over the Tropic of Cancer in the Northern Hemisphere. The sun has traveled to its farthest point north, and so the length of time between sunrise and sunset is the longest of the year.

In December, the sun is in the Southern Hemisphere, directly over the Tropic of Capricorn. The sun is farthest south, and the length of time between sunrise and sunset is the shortest of the year.

Southern Hemisphere

Winter and summer solstices are exchanged: Summer is December 22 and winter is June 21.

Equinox

The equinoxes occur in springtime during the month of March and in the fall during September. With each equinox, the center of the sun is directly above the earth's equator. At these two times, night and day are about the same length because the sun is crossing the equator. The sun is at an equal distance from the North and South Poles.

March 21 is the beginning of a long period of sunlight at the North Pole, as the sun crosses the equator and moves northward.

September 22 is the beginning of a long period of sunlight at the South Pole, as the sun crosses the equator and moves southward.

I decided to use the cyclical rhythms of solstice and equinox as a framework for you to design a personal Yoga practice using this book as a guide. Practicing Yoga in harmony with this 365-day rhythm increases your benefits.

I chose the particular Yoga sets and meditations for this book to better connect you to the rhythm of the earth's rotation cycles in relationship to the sun, thereby deepening your experience of interconnectedness with the environment and all of life. Each section of the book corresponds to the quality of naturally occurring energy and explains how to use it for your practice.

Breath control, central to Yoga practice, brings oxygen, awareness and prana into the body. Prana was described by ancient sages as the vibratory power that underlies all manifestation. The sun, earth, planets, moon, people, thoughts, emotions, animals, insects, and anything that can be imagined, seen or felt is a manifestation of One Source vibratory power. Thus, there is no power in things and nothing can make itself, but all things are manifestations of or made by the One Source. One Source animates or flows through everything. The flow of One Source energy is especially powerful during solstice and equinox.

my practice

Call it by any name, God, Self, the Heart or the seat of consciousness, it is all the same. The point to be grasped is this, that Heart means the very core of one's being, the centre, without which there is nothing whatever.

— Sri Ramana Maharishi[4]

After more than 25 years, my Yoga and meditation practice continues to be a source of delight and wonder for me. The Yoga flows, I witness my breath and I witness the posture and movement. Witnessing my meditation practice is *just this* or present moment awareness.

Occasionally, and certainly when I was just beginning to practice Yoga, my practice will start out dull and heavy. I feel stiff and inflexible. I am in my head and running the monkey mind of egoic thinking. The negative mind roars on and on, saying things like, "This is dumb" or "I don't need this" or "I want to quit!" I rarely quit, but usually in these practices where I start out with resistance, I do continue, and the positive mind will chirp in and say, "This isn't so bad" or "You are pretty good at this" or "Look at me!" After a bit of this, things tend to settle down, and from the neutral mind, I move as the peace of the Witness. My mind becomes still, even as thoughts come and go; my mind is still, even with sounds of a ringing phone or a honking truck or with the feeling of numbness in my leg. It has never failed; if I stick with my practice, I am always Witness. The Neutral Mind, Present Moment Awareness, call it what you like, but it is always there. Always.

When I teach or practice Kundalini Yoga, a wonderful thing happens. We always tune in using the Adi Mantra[5]: Ong Namo Guru Dev Namo, which is chanted at least three times. Everyone needs to do this before practicing Kundalini Yoga to connect to a line of transmission called the *Golden Chain*.

By tuning-in with the Adi Mantra and practicing Kundalini Yoga, we are connecting to a rich legacy, which is complete in its own structure beyond any individual. This gives us leverage for the power to change and make a difference in our lives. The Golden Chain is a line of transmission and history. Chanted for centuries, it is non-dual present moment awareness; the awareness from which we launch our practice, and share with others.

This means we welcome the generative, creative force of life, here, now, in our practice. We welcome that invisible teacher within, the radiant wisdom stored in our auras. We welcome and become a link in the Golden Chain of saints and sages who have practiced for centuries. What a gift!

It always happens that as a teacher, once I tune in with a class, I am teaching as Witness consciousness. I have taught several classes a week now for more than 7 years (more than 4,000 hours of teaching), and I teach each class as Witness consciousness. Intuitively, I know what to teach, and my students often shake their heads and say, "How did you know?"

To show you what I mean, I'll give a recent example. Walking up the stairs at home, to get dressed for teaching, I just knew that I had to change the class I had prepared. I would instead teach the Basic Spinal Series. I did wonder why for a moment because the series is an easy beginning (though very powerful) set, and this class had some intermediate and advanced Yogis in it. Once I arrived at the class, it became apparent why I knew to teach this set: A returning student, who has one leg and had not been to class for many months, brought a first time student, who is blind, to class. The Basic Spinal Series is done completely on the floor, with no standing postures, and has lots of meditative transition between each exercise — posture and then rest, posture and then rest. The postures are easy to explain without demonstration — no need to look at the teacher. It served as a wonderful introduction for a blind beginner and a great refresher for the rest of the class. How did I know to change my plan? The neutral mind or present moment awareness opens space for wisdom and intuition to just download on the spot.

when to practice

Any time. That said, the amrit vela is considered by Yogis to be the most beneficial time when the angle of the sun shines at 60 degrees upon the earth. This occurs at approximately 4 a.m. and 4 p.m. Choosing a time and rhythm that works for your life supports your practice. Keep it real! Daily practice is called *sadhana*.

Begin where you are. Your practice will vary and depend upon a variety of factors including if you have small children and if you are married or single, working or not working, a primary caregiver for a loved one, ill, or traveling. Simply notice what your practice looks like and be with it, noticing. Wahe Guru!!

Parenting is a full time spiritual practice. Yoga will cultivate your ability to be present for your children, which is all they really want or need from you, because then everything you give and receive flows to them from the wisdom and grace of the present moment. It is a gift for your children to participate with you or for them to know that you are practicing Yoga.

Committing to a relationship is a full time spiritual practice. Yoga practice will cultivate your ability to see and be seen, dissolving illusion and self-projection. You then have the awareness to end violence in your relationships, both with self and others. There is no *someone else*.

Being single is a full time spiritual practice. Practicing Yoga will cultivate your ability to experience relatedness, ending the feeling of separation. Your practice may bring you to the sacred marriage or union with your inner husband or wife.

Grieving from death or divorce is a full time spiritual practice. Yoga can help you to be present to any sadness, anger, loneliness, or fear and deliver you to an awareness that brings the *peace that passeth all understanding.*

Whatever life situation you find yourself in is a full time spiritual practice. Practicing Yoga can deliver you to Grace. Practicing may transform suffering into blessing.

getting started

Prepare[6] as if you are meeting your beloved because you are. Practice to remember and experience union with your finite and infinite self, I-I. Surrender through your heart to the Divine Shakti, allowing the universe to do the rest. To make yourself ready for practice and to enhance Kundalini Yoga, I offer the following :

1. Take a cold shower in the morning before you do Kundalini Yoga. If this is not possible, wash your hands, arms, face and neck with cold water. In other words, get cold water wherever you can and remember to briskly massage these areas! Whether your shower is indoors or outdoors, avoid taking a hot shower! Cold water is beneficial to your health. However, do not allow cold water to stream onto your genital area, stomach or thighs because it will leach out important minerals and warmth from these vital areas. It is the femur bone in the thigh that controls the calcium-magnesium balance in the body, so keep your thighs out of the direct stream of cold water!

   The cold temperature of the water on the rest of your body causes blood to rush from the interior organs to the surface of the skin. Your body will then feel warm because your capillaries carrying blood have opened to their maximum. When capillaries open up for increased blood flow, all deposits and toxins are cleaned out. When the capillaries return to normal, a fresh supply of blood then fills your inner organs, giving vitality for the day ahead. Your body has met the cold with its own circulatory power. Your skin will glow and you will have empowered your own health!

   Before you shower, massage oil onto your dry skin, head to toe. Allow the cold water to stream onto your feet, bottoms and tops, your body and your face. Starting with extremities, briskly rub your skin paying attention to lymph nodes under your arms to help prevent colds. Once the cold water feels warm, lather up! Sing or chant in the shower for inspiration and to keep yourself going. To end, towel dry, giving a vigorous self-massage.

2. Wear loose, comfortable, natural fiber clothing[7].

3. When indoors, make your space sacred by practicing in a clean, quiet place. Choose an object such as a flower, candle, picture of a saint or loved ones, or sacred book as a visual reminder that you are a spiritual being in a physical body having a human experience of joy.

4. Practicing Yoga outside, weather permitting, will deepen your experience and understanding of the postures such as Rock, Tree, Dog, and Mountain. As separation dissolves, feel the aliveness in nature as the aliveness in your body. Make sure the ground or blankets beneath you provide the padding you need. The beach is a wonderful place to do Yoga, especially at 4 a.m.

5. Use natural fibers when available for the following items: a mat or sheepskin, cushion, blanket, shawl, and head covering for meditation. A shawl or baseball cap work just fine to cover your head! Kundalini Yoga meditations generate a lot of spiritual heat which is released at the top of your head or crown chakra. Keep this heat, cover your head and bathe your aura with it. This is self-healing energy. Keep it; you earned it!

yoga kriyas

Evidence of Yoga practice and meditation can be traced through history as early as 1800 BC. Ancient scrolls from Tibet refer to Yoga and meditation being practiced over 40,000 years ago. A Yogi of great vision, Patanjali[8], lived somewhere between *AD 200 – AD 800* in India during the Classical Epoch. Today, we refer to Patanjali as the Father of Yoga because of his important work called the *Yoga Sutras,* which were the first written accounts of ancient oral traditions of Yoga and meditation. *Sutra* means *thread* and there are 195 sutras/aphorisms that, to this day, are considered the definitive overview of philosophy, goals and structure of Yoga and meditation.

Patanjali's Yoga Sutra (2.46)
Sthira sukham asanam
May the posture be steady and comfortable.

Kriya[9] means *completed action*. Kriya is an important part of the Kundalini Yoga as taught by Yogi Bhajan. It's a precise technology using pranayam (breath), asana (posture), mantra (sacred resonant sounds, silent, whispered, spoken, or chanted), and rhythmic movement. Do not eliminate postures or substitute one posture for another. When a posture is not appropriate for your body or health, modify with common sense. You can ultimately keep your body safe from injury by sitting or lying down with a straight spine and visualizing the posture using the specified breath and mantra for the designated time. This will work for you and will not upset the flow of energy and effect produced by the kriya. Really! *May the posture be steady and comfortable!*

Kriyas are always done exactly as written, with no exceptions, to safely achieve the maximum, desired effect. Respect the power of this technology. You may adjust the length of time for each posture or meditation, but never exceed the maximum time given. It is very important to keep it real. Do not move beyond your reach! Do not hold back! Remember to notice how you are doing what you are doing and remember who is noticing. With awareness, always move with compassion and surrender from the heart.

practicing

If you already have a consistent Yoga and meditation practice, please do your current practice either before or after you practice Kundalini Yoga. Don't intermingle them.

The Yoga sets and meditations can be used to create and sustain a practice that best meets the reality of your life now. Begin where you are, taking into consideration day, season and ability. The Yoga sets are divided into four sections corresponding to the four seasons and use Kundalini Yoga kriyas and meditations.

Warming-up Before a Kriya[10]

Yogi Bhajan, when leading Kundalini Yoga kriyas, usually did not use warm-ups, although he acknowledged that in some instances warm-ups are useful. Here are some options to choose from if you decide to include a warm-up before practicing a Kundalini Yoga kriya:

- Pranayam sequences are especially good for waking up the body and opening the lungs.
- Do a few repetitions of the short version of Sun Salutations (Surya Namaskara) included in the warm-up section of this book.
- You may choose to practice Spinal Flex, Cat-Cow and Life Nerve Stretches, all of which can stand alone, or can be used as a warm-up series. All of these are included in the warm-up section.

Author's note: Warm-ups can prepare your body for Kundalini Yoga kriyas because they improve your circulation, increase the flow of prana and release tension. Bringing your awareness to the connection between your breath and your body's movement will enhance your practice and bring you to the present moment.

Warming, stretching and energizing muscles, nerves, connective tissue, and spine prepares your body and prepares your hips and legs for sitting. Sun Salutations are excellent for warming-up and so are Spinal Flexes, Frog, Shoulder Shrugs and Life Nerve Stretches. Always make sure when warming up to work from the lower chakras to the higher chakras (or lower body to upper body) and balance front-bending exercises with back-bending exercises. Warm-ups and meditations can be done on their own.

Reminder: Warm-ups are separate from a kriya! Always maintain the integrity of sets as they were taught by Yogi Bhajan. Never add or subtract anything!

Practicing the Kriyas

Each season/section lists two kriyas, a meditation and a chanting meditation. Here are five possible ways to use each season:

1. Begin during the season that is current in your life. Use a kriya and meditation, in that order, and practice every day to receive full benefits. Do not exceed times given. Practicing every day is called *sadhana* and is considered by Yogis the most powerful way to access the Now.

2. Choose to do a kriya and/or meditation depending on the quality you want to invoke, regardless of the current season. For example, if you have a big presentation to prepare for work or school, you may decide to use a kriya and meditation from the spring section. Spring uses kriyas that stimulate the intellect for clarity of thought and the vocalization of ideas.

3. Consider doing one kriya and/or meditation each month of the season, whether you practice every day or once a week. You will deepen your experience of the kriya/meditation by repeating it.

4. Choosing one kriya and/or meditation and practicing it for three months every day will give you powerful results. A good meditation will break your old patterns by provoking your subconscious

to release any thoughts and emotional patterns that hinder you. To master the effects of Yoga or meditation, practice every day as *sadhana*. Habit controls us so much that it is said that we can actually change our destiny by changing our habits. According to Yogic science, the human mind works in cycles. You can use various cycles to replace unwanted patterns of behavior (mental or emotional habits) with a new more positive one. Commit to a particular meditation or kriya for a specific time[11]:

- It takes 40 days to change a habit.
- It takes 90 days to confirm the habit.
- In 120 days, the new habit is who you are.
- In 1,000 days, you have mastered the new habit.

5. Allow your practice to be a creative work in process. As you open your heart and reconcile your formless witness with your personal self, you see that you are like no one else and that you are part of a great love that knows no separation. Design your practice and experience!

body locks to seal energy

When your posture is correct, your body releases stress and relaxes so that you can become the posture and experience present moment awareness. Using the body locks called *bandhas* protects the alignment of your spine and projects your energy where you want it to go. Each body is different, so much so that some body-types will find one posture effortless and another body-type will find the same posture challenging. Using the body locks will protect every body. Remember that we are not striving for perfection, and bone structure and joints vary with each individual. You want to use correct alignment and discover what is real for your body, keeping steady and comfortable in the postures.

Bandhas: Root Lock, Neck Lock, Diaphragm Lock, and The Great Lock

Root Lock or *Mulbandh*

To apply Mulbandh[12], squeeze and lift the pelvic floor up and draw the navel point in. The navel point center is etheric, located a few inches down from the navel and in front of the lower spine.

To squeeze and lift the pelvic floor, you first contract the anus and hold, then contract the sex organ and hold. Last, pull in and up on the navel point.

All Yoga starts with the navel point because all Yoga movement begins at the navel point. To locate yours, place three fingers pointing horizontally under your belly button. Your navel point is just below your ring finger about 1 ½ inches below your belly button and in the transverse muscles. The Upanishads, a continuing genre of sacred Hindu literature dating as far back as the middle of the second millennium BCE up to our current century, says this about the navel center:

> In the center of the stomach, the navel center reposes in the chakra known as Manipura. Between the navel and the last bone of the spinal column is the Navel Point, shaped like a bird's egg. This encloses within itself the starting point of 72,000 nerves, of which 72 are vital and of these 72 there are 10 that are the most important. In order to have proper control over these nerves, one has to take special pains[12A].

In Mulbandh, the navel point is pulled in and up towards the spine, which causes the pelvis to rotate, pulling the sacrum down and lengthening the lower spine. Holding this alignment protects your lower spine during exercise. You will feel the tailbone moving down towards the floor when sitting or standing and using the Mulbandh.

Do not practice Mulbandh if you have high blood pressure, vertigo, high inter-cranial pressure, or amenorrhea. Pregnant women and women on the first day of their monthly cycle should not use Mulbandh. If you are not sure whether this lock is appropriate for you, please consult your doctor.

Neck Lock or *Jalandhar Bandh*

Root Lock and Neck Lock, when used together, lengthen and protect your spine and better distribute prana (life-giving energy) to be absorbed throughout your body.

First, pull in on your navel to anchor your pelvis. Then, to apply the Neck Lock[13], lift your chest, pull your chin in to straighten the natural backward curve of your neck towards the wall (or tree) behind you. You do not drop the chin to the chest. The chest rises to meet your chin, which is drawn in. Relax your shoulders and upper back and drop your shoulders down your back. This opens your heart to keep you from compressing your lower back.

In every Yoga posture, unless otherwise specified, use the Neck Lock. Applying the Neck Lock should not obstruct your flow of breath. Neck Lock elongates the spinal cord, bringing energy to the stem of the brain and providing a platform of support between the navel and the heart. Your head is balanced over your heart. Chin in, chest out opens the heart and supports your head correctly on your spine, allowing neck muscles to refrain from tensing up. Opening your heart opens your awareness. Create a pathway that allows your heart to lead your awareness to the Now.

If you do not use the Neck Lock, your flow of energy is blocked and unhealthy pressure can build up in your heart, behind your eyes, in your inner ear, and in your brain. The resulting stress will narrow your field of awareness.

Diaphragm Lock or *Uddiyana Bandh*

To breathe deeply, your diaphragm must expand downward on the inhale and upward on the exhale. Diaphragm Lock[14] stretches the muscles between the ribs so the rib cage can expand. This is an advanced practice and is not required for the Yoga sets in this book. When all three locks, Root, Neck and Diaphragm, are used, it is called the Great Lock.

To practice the Diaphragm Lock, sit on the heels or stand. If you are standing, keep your legs apart a little with your hands resting on your knees or a little above them. Sometimes people find it easier to learn this lock while lying on their backs.

To apply Uddiyana bandh, bend your torso forward, lifting the chest and keeping the neck aligned. Exhale as deeply and fully as you can. Hold your breath out and pull your chin in to seal your throat. This will create a vacuum in your chest so that you can suck your thoracic diaphragm upward making a hollow space under your ribs. (You will feel this suction also drawing the skin inward at the base of the throat in the notch of the sternum.) As the diaphragm lifts upward, the abdominal muscles can stay relaxed and just go along for the ride.) Hold your breath out as long as you comfortably can. Before you inhale, relax the tension, lower your diaphragm, and then inhale gently. Practice 1-5 minutes daily to develop your ability to do Diaphragm Lock.

Diaphragm Lock is difficult to practice if your abdominal muscles are tense. It must be practiced on an empty stomach and is only used after a complete exhalation with the breath held out. Do not practice Diaphragm Lock if you have high blood pressure, hernias or ulcers. Avoid during pregnancy and menstruation. As always, please consult a doctor if you are not sure an exercise is appropriate for you.

The Great Lock or *Mahabandh*

The Great Lock[14A] is the application of all three locks simultaneously with the breath held out. It is practiced after *pranayama* and exercise. It is done in various postures and combined with different mudras. It is part of the central infrastructure of Kundalini Yoga. Each student must master all the bandhas.

With all the locks applied, the body is in a perfect healing state. The practice and perfection of this lock is said to cure many ailments: improper blood pressure, menstrual cramps, poor circulation, irregularity, nocturnal emissions, and excessive preoccupation with fantasy. The glands, nerves and chakras are rejuvenated.

breath (pranayam)

Pranayam[15] is the science of breath, controlling the movement of prana through the use of breath techniques. Yogi Bhajan taught that:

> *The main problem in the world is stress. It is not going to decrease – it is going to increase. If through* pranayam *the shock can be harnessed, the entire stress and disease can be eliminated.*[15A]

Pranayam means *breath control*. Breath control has three parts: inhalation, retention and exhalation. By controlling the breath, you become conscious of the breath, which brings you to awareness of the Self, I-I and the present moment.

You can think of your brain as the hardware of your soul. When your breath is conscious and uses rhythmic repetition, you actually change your brain states. Simple repetition works the nervous system and secretes protein in the brain, changing brain chemistry so that your sensory capacity changes. Instead of being reactive you are able to accurately access information. Consciously directing the breath will control the flow of prana.

Your mind follows the breath all of the time! Consciously changing breath frequency[16] does affect the mind. Normally, people breathe at a rate of 16–20 breaths per minute. When you consciously breathe for 8 breaths per minute, you will feel relaxed and enjoy increased mental awareness and relief from stress. Breathing at a rhythm of 4 breaths per minute will automatically bring your mind to a meditative state. In addition, enhanced clarity of vision and heightened sensitivity in your body will be experienced while accessing your intuition due to stimulation of the pituitary and pineal glands.

When breathing is not controlled or conscious, a chain reaction happens. When breathing is fast, shallow and unconscious, the obedient mind responds and narrows its field of awareness. Racing thoughts, repetitive thoughts and scenarios, which are also called monkey mind, result. Finally, the body responds and tenses, bracing itself in protect mode, releasing chemicals within to support survival. When real danger is present, this release is a good thing. But when our breathing is unconscious, fast and shallow or paradoxical (Paradoxical breathing is breathing backwards. On the inhale, the belly goes in and on the exhale, the belly goes out- not good.), the responding mind puts stress on our nervous system and immune system. If this is prolonged, it exhausts the body's vitality.

As far as the body is concerned, there is only Now. Therefore, the body translates stressful thoughts as *Dangerous or stressful situations are really happening now!* Always, the breath affects the mind, and the mind affects the body, 100% of the time. Breathing consciously cultivates the flow of prana, the life-giving energy-juice, into your awareness. You then live life consciously and spontaneously instead of automatically and reactively.

To make your breath conscious during Yoga postures, open through the heart and use the mantra *Sat Nam* (unless otherwise directed). Mentally vibrate *Sat* on the inhale and *Nam* on the exhale. Let your breath and the mantra lead the movement for each exercise. *Sat Nam* means *true identity*.

practicing pranayam

Pranayam is an effective way to become conscious of your breathing to affect your emotions and thoughts, Now. Practice every day as needed, on or off the Yoga mat.

Long Deep Breathing in Three Parts[17]

I like to think of the three parts of the breath, (inhalation, retention and exhalation) as corresponding to three Hindu gods, Brahma the *Creator,* Vishnu the *Sustainer,* and Shiva the *Liberator* because this deepest of breaths opens the pathways for Shakti, the dynamic creative power of existence, to be present in your practice as an open heart. The Yoga-Vasishtha (3.13.31) tellingly defines prana as the "vibratory power" (*spanda-shakti*) that underlies all manifestation.

1. Sit or lie down with a straight spine protected by the Root Lock and Neck Lock (page 15). Begin inhaling from the bottom of the lungs, expanding the lower belly out. (Be sure not to expand your belly out too much or you will compress your spine.) Feel the breath directed to the lower sacrum, up the lower back and into the front and back of your lower rib cage.

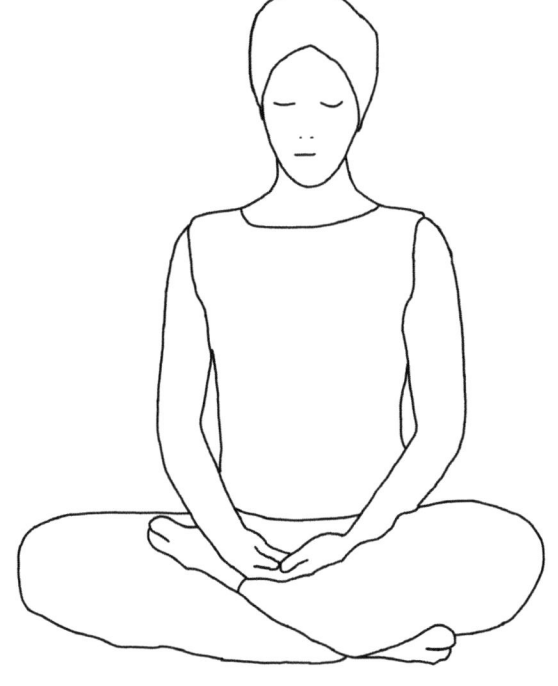

Three Part Breathing

2. Allow the breath to fill your lungs, expanding your ribcage in all directions up towards your shoulder blades. Feel your breath moving up your spine.

3. As you continue inhaling, your upper chest is filled to capacity. Your shoulder blades will spread apart and your chest and collarbones will lift.

4. To exhale, reverse the process, deflating first from the upper region, then the middle and finally the lower region. Notice how you feel. Repeat.

Breath of Fire

Breath of Fire[18] is a continuous balancing breath. Equal on the inhale and exhale, your breath is a kind of flutter between your navel and solar plexus. It is stimulating and relaxing at the same time because the rhythms of the heart and breath move at different rates. Once you get the hang of it, 120-180 breaths per minute is a good classic rhythm. If that is too fast, you may start slower.

1. To properly learn how to maintain the rhythm, sit with a straight spine, open your mouth, stick out your tongue and pant like a dog. This works every time. Once you have the rhythm, continue the breath now with your mouth closed, breathing through your nose.

2. Sit with a straight spine. Open through your heart as the chest lifts. Relax your face. Relax your shoulders. Beginning with the rhythm that is appropriate for you, inhale and exhale equally through your nose. Breathe from the diaphragm with your focus at the solar plexus and it will feel like a flutter. Breath of Fire should feel relaxing and nearly effortless. Your navel point is naturally and softly drawn in and up on the exhale and naturally and softly drawn down and out on the inhale. Think up and down rather than in and out.

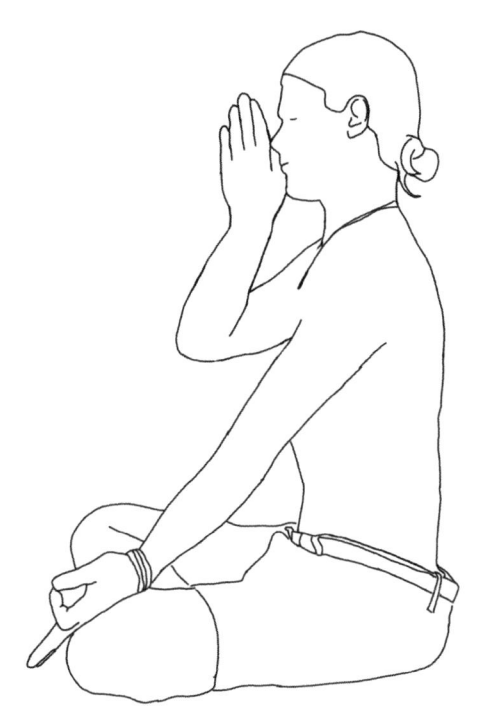

Left and Right Nostril Breathing

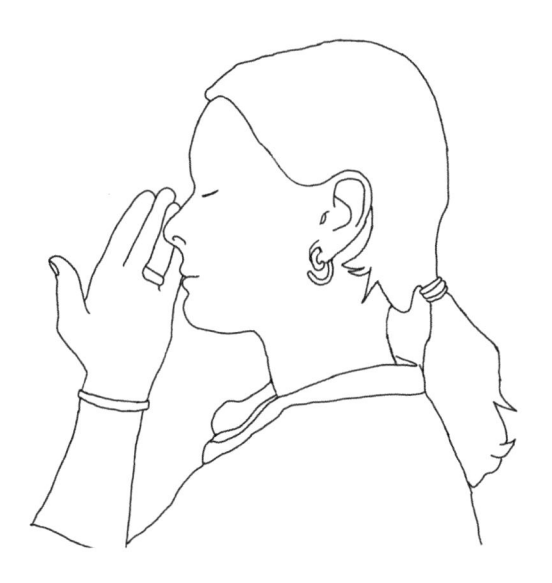

Every 2 1/2 hours, we experience a change in our natural breathing cycle. The breath is dominant in either the left or the right nostril.[19] Check it out right now. Block one nostril as you breathe and then switch to blocking the other. One side will be breathing stronger than the other. Breathing more from the left nostril is relaxing. Breathing more from the right nostril is energizing. Breathing equally from both nostrils creates a feeling of balance. If you need to finish a deadline for work in a hurry and you are naturally breathing more from the left nostril, you can consciously direct the breath through the right nostril to give you energy, quickly and naturally. Sleeping while lying on your left side will produce more dreams because right nostril breathing is more active. If it's late at night and your mind is racing, left nostril breathing will relax you and help you get to sleep.

Nostril Breathing

Alternate Nostril Breathing[19]

1. Sit with a straight spine. Your left hand is resting on the left knee in Gyan Mudra (page 30).

2. Bend your right arm, keeping the upper arm close to the body. Block your right nostril with your right thumb, keeping your right fingers together and pointing them straight up. Inhale through the left nostril.

Alternate Nostril Breathing

23

3. Remove your thumb from the right nostril and pivot your right hand so that your ring finger or index finger blocks your left nostril. Exhale completely through your right nostril. Still blocking your left nostril, inhale through your right nostril.

4. Pivot your hand and block the right nostril with your right thumb. Exhale completely through your left nostril. Inhale deeply through your left nostril.

5. Block your left nostril and repeat this rhythm for one minute or longer.

Sitali Breath

Sitali Pranayam[20] is used to achieve a powerful cooling and relaxing effect on your body while maintaining alertness. It is used to aid digestion and lower fevers. At first, you may notice a bitter taste on the tongue. This is a result of detoxification and will pass. Your taste on the tongue will become sweet.

1. Sit with a straight spine. Curl your tongue into a U shape, if you are able.

2. Inhale through the curled tongue (or over your flat tongue if your tongue doesn't curl).

3. Exhale through the nose.

4. Repeat. Practice for one minute or longer.

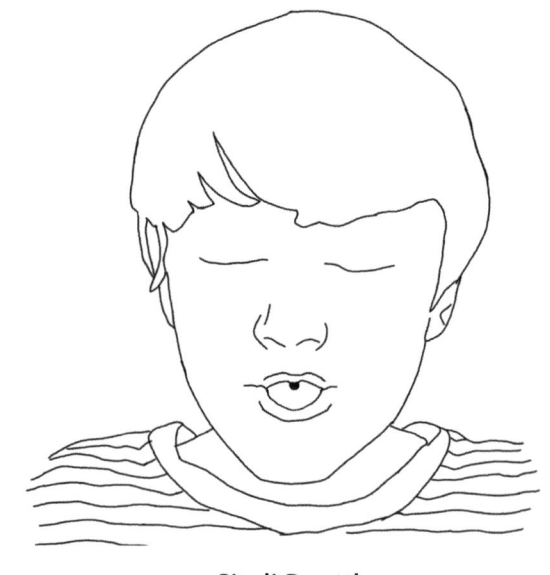

Sitali Breath

One Minute Breath

Kundalini Yoga uses pranayam and bandha (body locks) to bring you to present moment awareness. This state of stillness is called *shuniya* or *zero*. In stillness as zero, a new rhythm or pattern is created as Kundalini flows to change your universe. Breath frequency is how to affect your mind; in order to control the quality of your mind, you must be conscious and control the breath. By breathing one cycle per minute[21], you optimize cooperation between the two hemispheres of your brain and your whole brain is stimulated. Your intuition will develop and you will enjoy a dramatic relaxation and calming of anxiety, fear and worry.

1. Sit with a straight spine. Through your nose, inhale long, slowly and deeply, allowing 20 seconds to inhale.

2. Hold your breath for 20 seconds. Your face is relaxed and there is no tension in your chest.

3. Allow 20 seconds to exhale through your nose.

4. Repeat two more times and gradually build up your time.

Suspending the Breath

Suspending the breath[22] means that you relax the muscles of your diaphragm, ribs and abdomen that are responsible for the constant motion of your breath. The goal is a switch in your metabolic activity, a balancing of your nervous system and emotional control. It is not simply holding the breath! You must remain aware of your posture and mindful of your breath while maintaining a straight spine and applying the Neck Lock. It is important to relax the neck and throat muscles and to soften your tongue. You will train your subconscious to remember how to breathe properly even when you are not fully alert.

Suspending on the Inhale

1. Inhale deeply, opening through your heart. Create a calm internal awareness and observe changes in your body and mind.

2. Bring your attention to the upper ribs and collarbone. Lift the upper ribs slightly and hold them in place.

3. Pull the chin in, become completely still and relax your shoulders, throat and face.

4. If you feel the urge to exhale, inhale a tiny amount instead.

Suspending on the Exhale

1. Begin with a complete exhale, keeping your spine straight. Create a calm internal awareness and observe changes in your body and mind.

2. Pull your navel point back towards the spine.

3. Lift the lower chest and diaphragm, relax and compress your upper ribs.

4. Pull the chin in, become completely still and relax your shoulders, throat and face.

5. If your muscles start a reflex to inhale, consciously exhale a little more.

mantra

In the West, we are not accustomed to using sound deliberately for healing and awareness. The multi-billion dollar music industry, however, knows the power of sound to affect you. Someone once said, "Rock and roll brought the Iron Curtain down." Music has narrowed the generation gap, uniting young and old, and music powerfully lives in our collective psyche. Popular music has become the mantra of the West, and you know firsthand the power of a song to change your mood.

The chanting[23] meditations in each section are an opportunity for you to experience the precision of sound rhythms or *naad*[24]. Yogi Bhajan, whose PhD was in communications, described naad during his November 24, 1990 lecture in Hamburg, Germany.

> Effective communication is called naad — harmonious speaking and hearing at the same time — something which connects. Ordinarily, people do not have harmonious understanding or hearing or listening. Nor do people have the clarity of speaking. So what we are doing within the smallness of us is unpredictable because we do not know what we are saying or if what is heard is understood or not . . . We are a simple, living, human being, and we should watch our living and hear our inner sound, which is pure love, pure life, pure existence.

The experience of precise rhythm, using sacred sounds, opens your Divine Heart, which is the One Heart that unites us all. Yogi Bhajan said that Heart makes you Universal. Chant with balance, grace and joy. As you feel your Heart open, let the universe do it for you! Let it flow. Connect as I-I. Notice. Just this.

Kundalini Yoga has a rich tradition of using mantra and sound to access the neutral mind or shuniya. Even as you experience stillness, all of physical reality is vibrating with sound at varying frequencies, 100% of the time! There are physical phenomena of sound and original primal sound, which created the physical universe. Scientists call this ever present primal sound vibration *cosmic radiation*.

Resonating the mantras, both silently and by chanting, brings you to a vibrant inner stillness. Using sound and mantra, you will release stress and create new neuron-pathways in the brain. You replace monkey mind thoughts with thoughts that create unity. As separations dissolve, healing happens. Then, as you live your life, you can respond with joy. Intuiting wisdom from your true identity, I-I, is an active, powerful and creative way to live. It is your human birthright.

mudra / hand positions

A mudra[25] is a hand position used in meditation to stimulate energy meridians in the palms or tips of the fingers and thumbs to activate the brain and nervous system. Each finger and each thumb represent a planet and the qualities associated with it. The word *mudra* translates to mean *seal*.

Thumbs represent the Earth or ego and manifestation.
Index fingers represent Jupiter and wisdom and expansion.
Middle fingers represent Saturn and emotion and patience.
Ring fingers represent the Sun and energy and health.
Pinky fingers represent Mercury and communication and power to relate.

Venus Lock
Author's Note: Venus Lock is opposite for men and women. Women: Interlock your fingers with the left thumb closest to your body and pressing into the fleshy mound at the base of the your right thumb. Men: Interlock fingers with your right thumb closest to your body and pressing into the fleshy mound at the base of your left thumb.

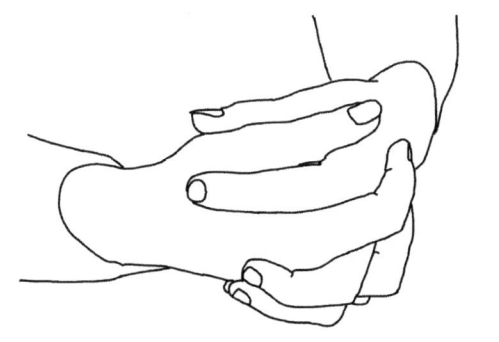

Sat Kriya Mudra

Author's Note: Interlace the fingers except for the index fingers, which point straight up. Men cross the right thumb over the left thumb; women cross the left thumb over the right.

Bear Grip Mudra

Author's Note: Bear Grip at the heart center. Clasping hands, your left palm faces out from chest, thumb on the bottom. Right palm faces chest with thumb on the top. Curl the fingers of both hands so they form a fist. Pull hard as if trying to pull hands apart so that forearms make a straight line.

Gyan Mudra

Author's notes: This Mudra is the same for both hands. Applying pressure to the tip of the thumb with the tip of the index finger stimulates energy meridians to activate your deepest wisdom. Fingers are straight.

Prayer Mudra

Author's notes: This universal gesture stimulates the thymus gland. Make sure thumbs are gently pressing the sternum and index fingers are touching thumbs. Feel an opening in your heart. Fingers point straight up.

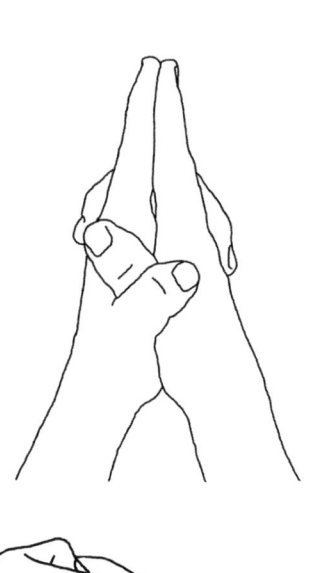

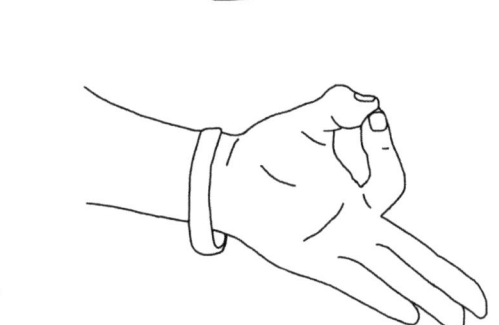

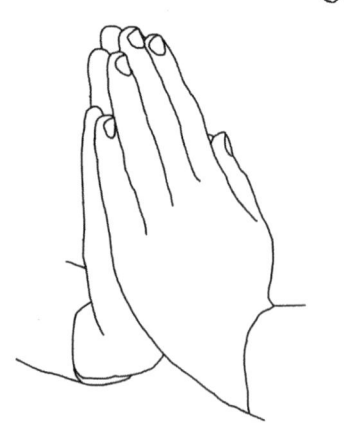

focal point for your eyes

Brow, Tip of the Nose, Chin, Crown, and 1/10th Open

During meditation and postures, many times you will use a focal point[26] or gaze called *drishti* to focus the mind. Drishti is any focal point that focuses the mind such as breath or chanting in addition to the focal points for your eyes.

Drishtis

Brow — *Shambavi Mudra* also called the third eye or *Ajna* chakra and is located at the root of your nose. Your attention is on the brow and your eyes are gently raised to gaze between the eyebrows and inward a little bit. This action stimulates the pituitary gland developing your intuition. Your central nerve force, *sushmuna* or most gracious channel, is stimulated. Sushmuna is the central conduit along the spinal column through which pran*a* or life force flows from the root chakra to the crown and the crown to the root. Wisdom gained by consciously moving prana through seven chakras is stored in your aura, which Yogi Bhajan called the eighth chakra.

Tip of the Nose — *Agiaa Chakra Bandh* or Lotus Point Meditation is the highest lock. It controls the mind, stimulating your pineal gland and your frontal lobe to create new energy pathways in your brain patterns. You are putting pressure on your optic nerve as you gaze at the tip of your nose, which stimulates the three energy currents:

1. Ida or channel of comfort, which is situated left of sushmuna, is associated with your inner Moon and terminates with the left nostril. It has a cooling effect on the body. Physically, it corresponds to the parasympathetic nervous system.

2. Pingala or tawny current, which is situated right of sushmuna, is associated with your inner Sun and terminates with the right nostril. It has a warming effect on the body. Physically, it corresponds to the sympathetic nervous system.

3. Sushmuna is the central channel and is stimulated to bring you to a center of balance. Called *form of delight,* it is said by Yogis to *devour time,* which is created by the Sun and the Moon, and you then win the immortal condition of self-realization. Always Now.

Chin is called the *Moon Center.* Your eyes are closed and rolled down towards the tip of your chin. You will see yourself clearly and this focal point brings cooling and calming.

Crown is located at the top of the head and is called the Tenth Gate or crown chakra. Your eyes are closed and rolled upwards as if looking through the top of your head. This energizes the crown chakra and stimulates the pineal gland.

1/10th Open or 9/10th closed, sometimes referred to as drunk eyes, is a focal point where your eyelids are light and relaxed and your eyes are unfocused. You will feel calm and develop equilibrium. By slightly stimulating your optic nerve, your system will stay open to the effects of the meditation.

meditation

I find that there's room in me for everything, everyone, every situation, every flavor of being. I love the openness that I am.[27]

— Byron Katie

There are three states of mind[28]: *sattva* or *beingness*, *tamas* or *darkness* and *rajas* or *affectedness*. A sattvic mind is crystallized like a gem and flawless. You are not fragmented by your reactions. A tamasic mind is slow, foggy and tired. You use poor judgment and are dull and confused. A rajasic mind is monkey mind. It jumps with erratic energy and it doesn't take much to send it in any direction.

Your mind is always creating. The goal of meditation is to control or re-direct the creativity of your life. You can cultivate the ability to choose the direction of your next thought; otherwise, unbidden thought can control the direction you take. Ask yourself, "Is life what it is or is life what I want it to be?" Identification with whatever thought pops into your head can cloak your experience of reality. We are connected to everything: past, future, movies, other people, events. We experience it all in the Now. Clarity of mind embracing the Now is *Buddhi Mind*.

The goal of meditation is not to simply create a nice place to be. Kundalini Yoga meditations clear out your subconscious fears and habits that do not serve you in a positive manner so you can hold up under pressure in real life. You get real! Your identification with egoic thoughts is replaced with your true self, connected to the infinite. When you meditate, you become still and notice the never-ending flow of thoughts. It is impossible to get rid of thoughts, but by noticing your thoughts and allowing them to be without judgment, they release you. Just notice. Just this. As your thoughts show up and leave, you notice that the whole world is in your mind, and your mind creates your perspective about life. Your ego identifies with thought and creates a false identity for yourself. A relaxed mind opens the heart and you direct thoughts to create a life as joy.

Your mind by itself has no power. Your mind is not a thing. Your mind is not just personal. Your mind is a process and that process is connected to everything. The process has great power but it has no reality. The process of the mind helps you to create your reality for your life. When you surrender through the heart, you relax and let go of egoic striving so that true creativity can happen. A relaxed mind is a creative mind. When your mind is totally relaxed and without stress, you experience your ability to access information through your intuition. You then accept or reject any thought from your deepest wisdom. You may access the universal mind, called *citta*. Meditation relaxes the mind so you can consciously direct your mind to create with joy. When your mind is relaxed, it does not mean that the mind is sleepy. It's exactly the opposite! Your mind is free to powerfully engage, think clearly and access your most dynamic thinking processes.

how to sit, stand and bend

Kundalini Yoga practice aligns all 10 bodies. That's right! Yogi Bhajan taught that we all have 10 bodies of which the physical body is just one. This section deals with the physical body. I explain all 10 bodies in the next section of this book.

Yoga postures depicted in the West have often been stylized by various media and are misleading. Photographs of people in *pretzel* poses are deceptive because they imply (and have set) a standard or goal of perfection that is exclusive! The models in popular Yoga magazines and manuals have been born with a bone structure that allows them a range of movement that is fashionable. Considered by Western media to be beautiful and correct, the range of movement that they enjoy and display is not necessarily the result of a better sadhana or Yoga practice.

Paul Grilley teaches that your flexibility is determined by two naturally occurring conditions: tension and compression. This is vitally important for you to understand if you are going to practice Yoga and maintain a Yoga practice that is alive and real, addressing your body and working with the bone structure with which you were born. It's easy to understand once you know what to look for.

You are not looking to duplicate another person's potential or limitations. Here's what you *do* look for: tension, which is muscular, and compression, which is where the bones at your joints meet. If your muscles are taut, they will not allow you to stretch into your full range of flexibility. Consistently practicing Yoga will work through all muscle tension over time and allow greater flexibility and range of motion. The amount of time needed varies from person to person. Once you have worked through tensile (muscular) limitations, you reach compression - where bone touches bone. At this point, you have reached your full range of motion and no amount of practice will increase your flexibility beyond this point. It is the range with which you were born! Practicing Yoga and stretching from your full range of motion and flexibility is enjoyable, is beneficial to your health, brings new bone growth, and creates strong bones. It feels great!

It's the bones you were born with that determine your range of motion. And every person's bones are put together differently. The length of your arms in relation to the length of your torso or the angle of the twist in your forearm or how your femurs connect to your pelvis will determine how you do various Yoga poses. Your bone structure informs you how to modify a pose when appropriate and, in some cases, *if* you can comfortably do certain Yoga poses! You work with what you were born with to enjoy and benefit from Yoga. We simply all look a bit different in the poses if our practice is alive and real. And two people who do look the same are not feeling the same!

Some people will never bring their chin to their chest because their bones compress (or touch), preventing them from opening any further. No amount of stretching or Yoga can change this. Some people will never place their heels flat on the floor in Triangle Pose (Downward Dog) unless they bring their feet far forward of the standard Yoga model's stance. And the decision to move the feet forward in order to make heels flat or to keep the feet placed further back with heels off the floor depends upon whether one decides to stretch the legs, ankles and feet or the spine, shoulders and arms. Some people can stretch and open both upper and lower portions of the body in Triangle Pose (Downward Dog) all at once, and some people must choose one or the other. Knowing where your bones compress in all of your major joints will give you the confidence to practice consciously and safely.

You will learn to feel the difference between compression (bones) and tension (muscles) by paying attention to where the sensations of stretch are occurring. If you feel discomfort at the joint, it is compression. If you feel discomfort in the muscle, it is tensile.[28A]

Seated Poses[29]

Easy Pose, Rock Pose, Half Lotus, Lotus Pose, Celibate Pose and Sitting In A Chair.

Most meditations and some Yoga postures call for sitting with a straight spine in Easy Pose. Compassion is *how* to sit, so keep it real; it's the only way not to cause injury to your body. Use a cushion or rolled up blanket to elevate the hips and support the spine or sit in a chair or lie down if that's the best way to achieve a straight spine.

Author's note: Meditating while sitting in Full Lotus or Celibate Pose is an advanced practice, and your bone structure plays a key factor in your ability and comfort in these postures. Never stretch beyond your edge! Beginners new to Yoga would benefit from attending a series of Yoga classes before attempting Full Lotus or Celibate Pose on their own.

How to Sit

If you are not accustomed to sitting with a straight spine on the floor, it is important that you make the following adjustment, raise your hips slightly by sitting on a natural fiber rug or sheepskin. A rolled up blanket or cushion also will do. Always sit with a curve in your lower spine without it being too curved inward and it should not curve outward. If your knees don't easily come close to the floor, place stacked blankets or cushions under your knees to provide support. This also helps support tight hips. Keep your feet active while in seated, bent-knee postures.

Author's note: Before attempting Full Lotus, warm ups should include a series of hip openers (page 75).

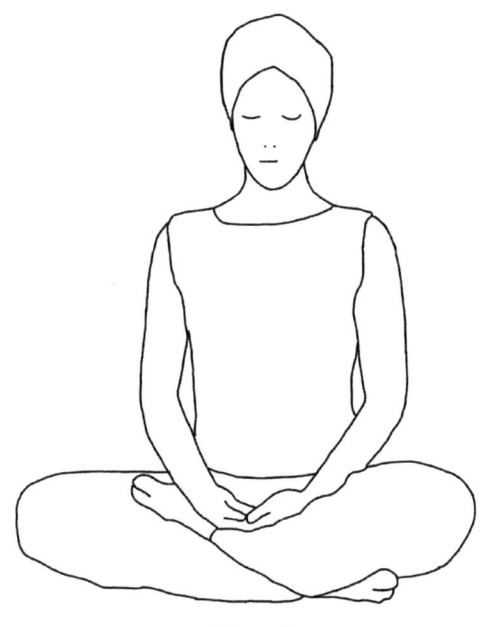

Easy Pose

Sit with a straight spine. Lift the heel of one foot up near the groin. Arrange the foot on top so it rests directly on the calf, with the ankle of the top foot about two inches up from the ankle of the bottom foot. In this pose, make sure to press the lower spine forward. It will have a tendency to slip backward.

If the previous posture is too strenuous, try this variation. Put one foot under the opposite knee and then draw the extended foot under the other knee. Pull the spine up straight and press the lower spine slightly forward.

Author's note: In Easy Pose, tilt your pelvis so that your tailbone moves towards the floor, lengthening your spine down. Gently lift your ribcage. Shoulders relax down the back. Chest out and chin in. Feel your heart open. The top of your head is flat, reaching towards the sky.

Author's modification: Rock Pose is a good modification for you to use in place of Easy Pose if you do not find Easy Pose easy!

Perfect Pose

This pose is excellent for stimulating the nervous system and utilizing your body's sexual energy. Once mastered, this posture automatically puts you into meditation.

Easy Pose

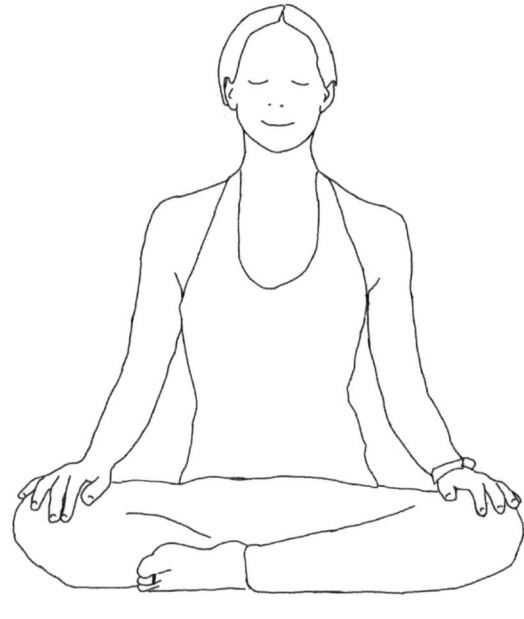

Easy Pose (Alternate)

To begin: Bring your left heel under your sex organ. Your left heel should touch the spot on the pelvis between the sex organ and the rectum. Bend your right leg and put your toes on the right foot behind the right knee. Your toes on your right foot are contained in the bend of the left knee. Only the big toe is exposed. Pull your spine straight.

Rock Pose

This posture is called *Rock Pose* because it is said that if you sit like this, you will strengthen your digestive system so well that you could digest rocks!

To begin: Sit on your heels, pull a light neck lock, keep the spine straight.

Author's notes: Keep the tops of your feet flat on the floor. Your heels will press onto nerves in the center of your buttocks, which aid digestion. Check your alignment: Spine is straight, ribcage gently lifts and shoulders relax down the back. Chest out and chin in. Feel your heart open. The top of your head is flat, reaching towards the sky.

Author's modification: Use pillows or blankets under your feet and/or between your calves and thighs for comfort.

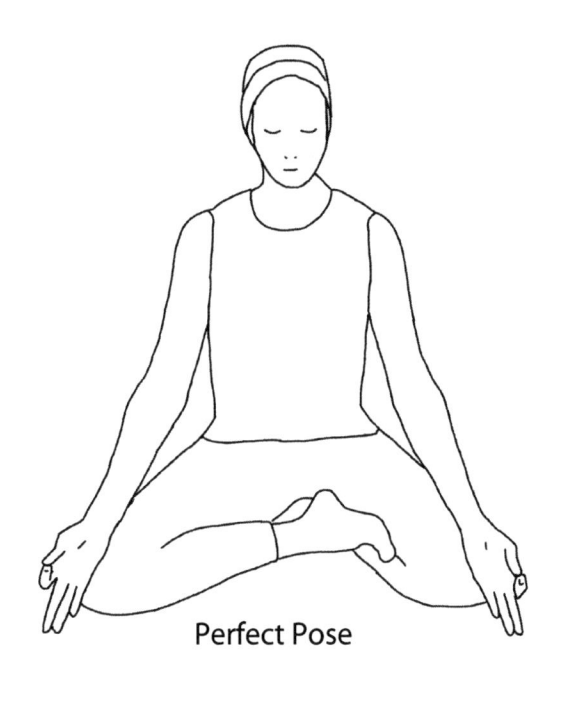

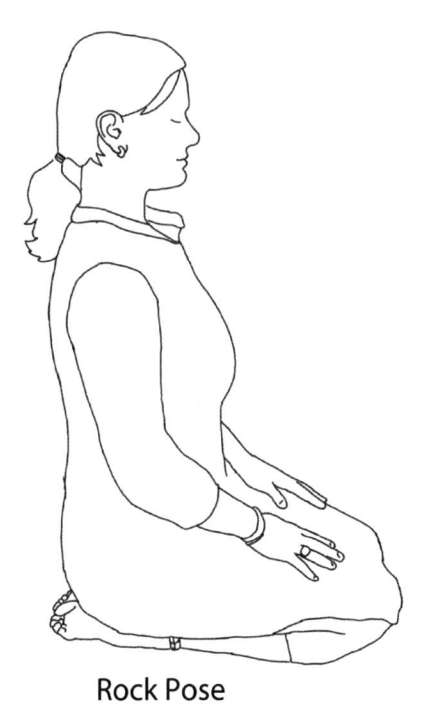

Perfect Pose

Rock Pose

Half Lotus Pose

Put the left foot into the groin so that the sole of the foot is against the uppermost part of the thigh. Place the right foot over the left ankle, so that it rests on the right thigh, sole of the foot turned up.

Author's note: Prepare by doing some hip openers (page 75).

Carefully grasp the underside of your left foot and ankle with both of your hands. Gently bring your left foot up into your right groin. Check your alignment and maintain a straight spine, chest up and shoulders relaxed. Open through your heart. Be sure to repeat on your other side for an equal amount of time to balance the opening of your hips. If your knees hurt, stop!

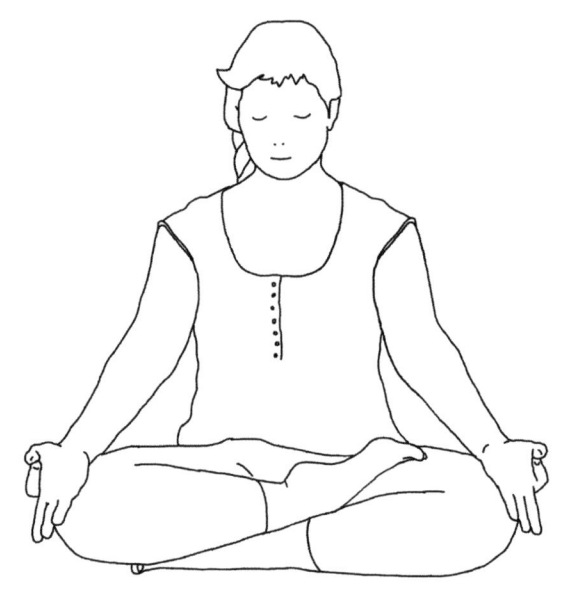

Half Lotus Pose

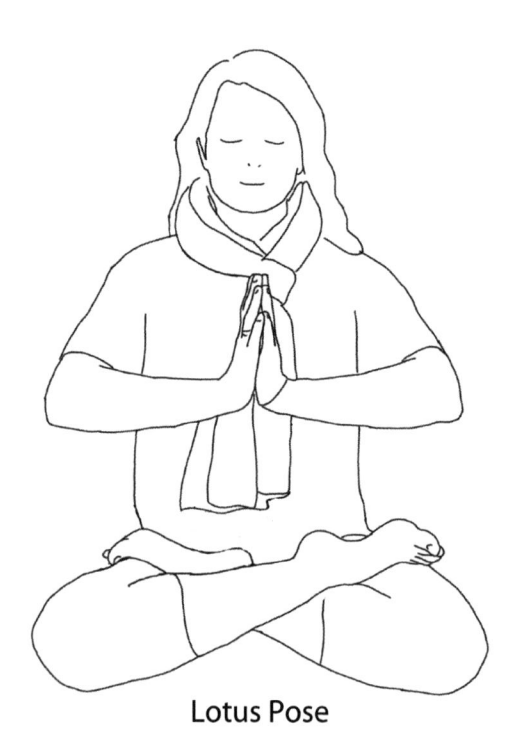

Lotus Pose

Lotus Pose is ideal for meditation, if you can do it comfortably, because it is extremely restful, improves circulation throughout your body and strengthens your back, improving posture. Full Lotus requires flexibility and rotation in your hips and ankles. There should be absolutely no discomfort in your knees. If your knees hurt, stop!

Bend the left leg so the left heel comes to the groin. Lift the left foot onto the upper right thigh. Bend the right leg so that the right foot goes over the left thigh, as close to the abdomen

Lotus Pose

as possible. Straighten the spine. Lift the chest and press the lower spine slightly forward. In this position you will feel locked in place. Once you are in it you can meditate very deeply and the position will maintain itself. There are very few exercises or meditations that require this posture, but it is recognized as one of the best asanas for deep meditation.

Author's note: Prepare by doing some hip openers (page 75) and then Half Lotus on each side.

Sit in Easy Pose with a straight spine. Allow the weight of your body to sink to the floor, grounding through your sit bones and perineum. Feel your connection to gravity. Feel rooted to the earth. Elongate your spine and open through your crown. Your ribcage floats up and away from your waist. Relax your shoulder blades down your back. Keep your navel moving in towards your spine.

Notice how you are doing what you are doing. Open through your heart. Breathe. To further prepare for Full Lotus, carefully grasp the underside of your left foot and ankle with both of your hands. Gently bring your left foot high onto your right thigh and up to your right groin. Carefully bring your right leg over your left leg and place your right foot into your left groin. Hold for a few seconds or longer. Uncross your legs and do the other side.

Celibate Pose

This posture is called Celibate Pose because sitting this way channels sexual energy by moving it from the lower chakras up the spine to your higher centers.

Begin by sitting on the heels. Spread the feet far enough apart so that your hips will fit between them. Move slowly, bending your knees and sitting down with your feet on either side of

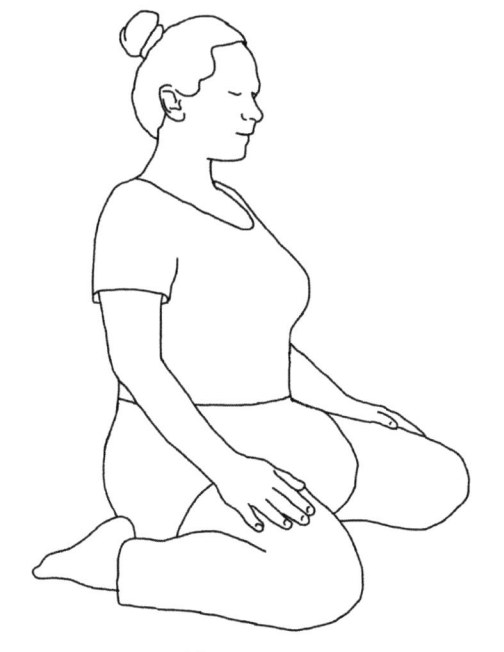

Celibate Pose

your hips. Try to maintain a straight spine. The flexibility should come from the hips, not the knees. This should not hurt the knees. If there is too much pressure on the knees, do not lower the buttocks all the way to the ground. Instead use a block or pillow under the buttocks.

Author's note: Check your alignment: Spine is straight, ribcage gently lifts and shoulders relax down the back. Chest out and chin in. Feel your heart open. The top of your head is flat, reaching towards the sky. There should be no discomfort in your knees. If your knees hurt, stop!

Author's modification: In a chair, sit with a straight spine, rooting your sit bones into the chair and keeping both feet flat and hip-width on the floor.

Sitting In A Chair

If none of the basic sitting poses are comfortable, you may sit in a straight-backed chair that gives you firm support. It is essential that the feet be equally placed on the ground ensuring that the lower spine and hips do not get out of balance, and that the blood distribution in the pelvic area will be balanced with respect to the two sides of the body. Keep the spine straight and the neck aligned.

Author's modification: Place a firm pillow or two under your feet if they do not reach the floor. Keep the spine straight and the neck aligned

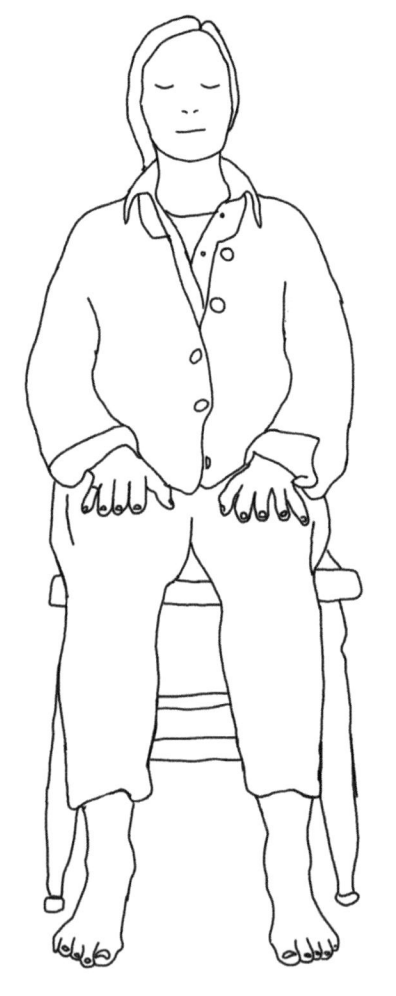

Sitting in Chair

Standing Straight (Mountain Pose)

Feet are your foundation! Properly aligned, you will build strength in ligaments that run along both sides of your legs and knees. To practice, stand up straight with your feet together, toes and heels touching, or with feet hip-width apart (Mountain Pose).

Author's note: Bone structures vary, and many people report preferring to stand with their feet hip-width apart versus feet together. Keep it alive and dynamic for you. Align your feet so that the second toes are parallel. Lift all 10 toes off the ground and press into the 4 corners of your feet (the bases of your big and little toe and inner and outer heel). Spread your toes, extending the big toe and the little toe in opposite directions. Keeping your toes spread, gently place each toe individually on the ground, maintaining awareness of your feet. (Maintain this awareness in any posture, standing or sitting, unless otherwise stated. For example, even if you are in a seated forward bend, the feet should remain active, as if you were standing on the ground). Now, with the inhale, feel the energy moving from deep within the earth, up through the base of your feet and flowing up your legs. Allow this flow of energy to rise to the navel point (about 2 inches below the belly button). Exhale and feel the energy flowing down from your navel point, down through your legs, through your feet and back into the earth. Repeat until you feel deeply rooted as a mountain.

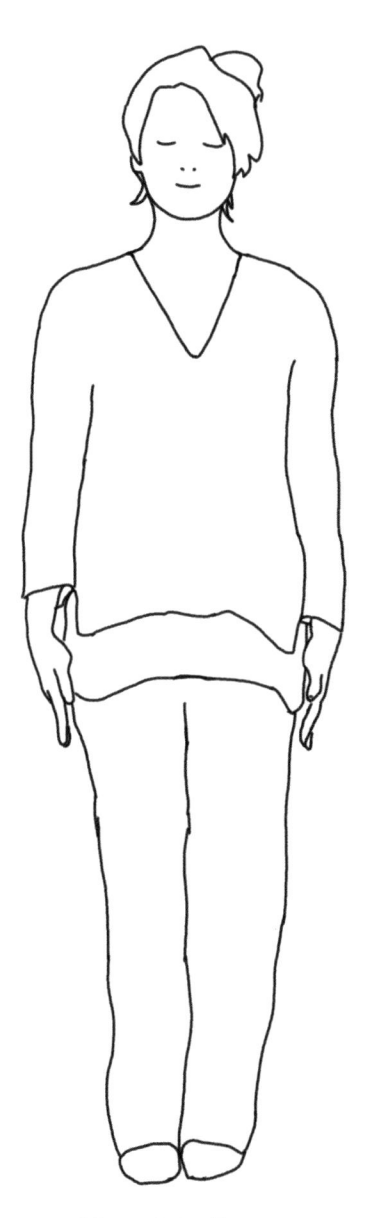

Mountain Pose

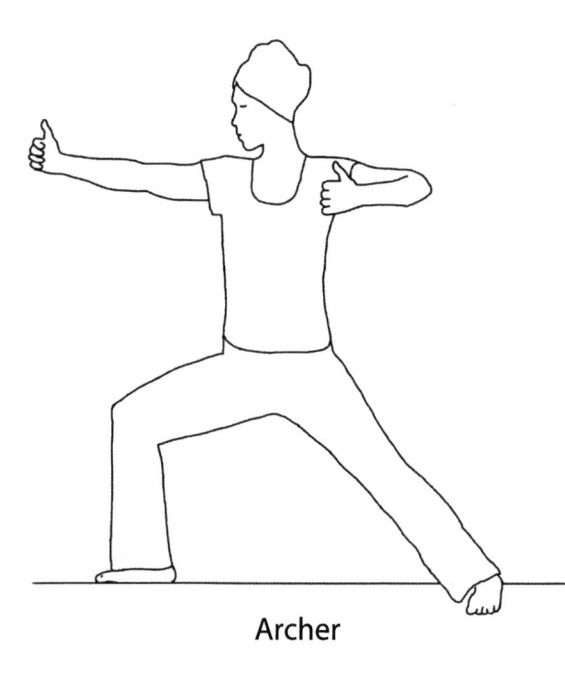

Knee Alignment: When a posture, such as Archer, Chair or Crow, calls for deep knee bends, make sure the posture is steady and comfortable! Protect your knees, keep them safe and bend with compassion!

Notice how you are doing what you are doing. What you do to yourself, you do to the rest of us. There is no *someone else*. If your ego is projecting ideas about perfection, competition and judging, that is the reminder to go more deeply into your breath and just this: Notice who is noticing.

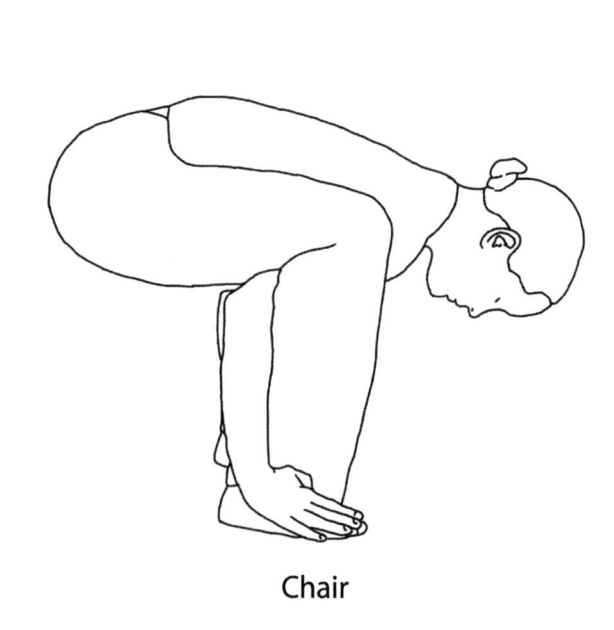

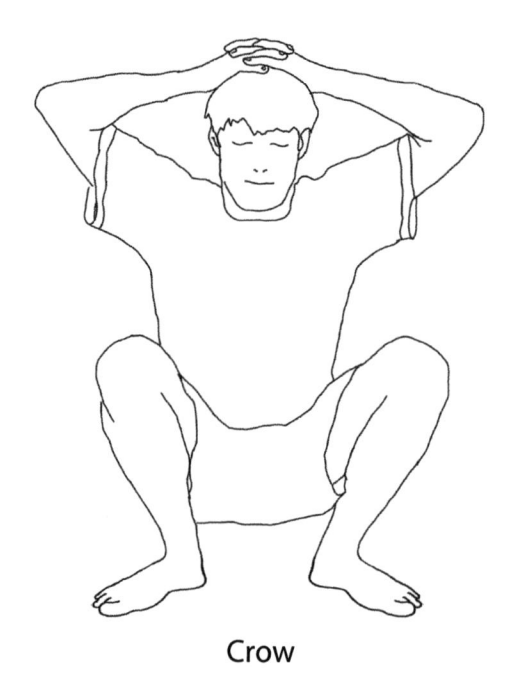

Archer

Chair

Crow

energy centers in the body

Precisely because the ego, the soul and the Self can all be present simultaneously, we can better understand the real meaning of egolessness, a notion that has caused an inordinate amount of confusion. But egolessness does not mean the absence of a functional self (That's a psychotic, not a sage.); it means that one is no longer exclusively identified with that self.

— Ken Wilber

Yogi Bhajan taught that we have eight chakras[31]. Seven energy centers or vortexes are within the body and one, called the aura, is outside of the body. These centers spin with energy to unite your consciousness—body, mind and spirit. Chakra expert, Anodea Judith, defines chakras as *centers of activity for the reception, assimilation and transmission of life energies.*

Physically, electromagnetic chakra activity can be measured to help diagnose and heal illness. Physical behavior and sensations can represent chakra activity such as *butterflies in the stomach* (third chakra) or *a frog in the throat* (fifth chakra). Your intuition and higher wisdom, such as knowing who is calling before you pick up the telephone, reside in the sixth and seventh chakras. Each chakra is a paradigm of consciousness that has prevailed in the world since the beginning of time. The Age of Aquarius is a time when many people will open through their heart into higher chakras as a stable state of consciousness.

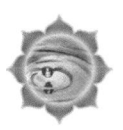

We have all had peak experiences of joy! These whiffs of euphoria can happen during meditation, while in pristine nature or when with loved ones, such as the birth of a child or while making love. Usually we quickly return to our everyday consciousness.

Living each moment as a state of joy is possible as a stable rather than a fleeting state of consciousness. When we commit to practicing Yoga consistently, we achieve an inner joy and create our life from upper triangle chakras (which intrinsically include and are supported by the lower triangle.) This is the essence of Grace shining through your heart.

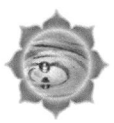

Yogi Bhajan gave us Kundalini Yoga so that we could learn to distinguish from what chakra we are speaking or from what chakra a person is listening to us. That understanding is the path to peace. You learn to see totality with compassionate clarity.

Projectivity in Kundalini Yoga balances the intelligence. Sometimes the psyche of intelligence is not balanced with the psyche around you. There are three psyches: your individual inner psyche, the psyche which is in your immediate environment and the psyche of the landscape, which is bigger, higher and wider. If these three psyches are not in balance, you are not in harmony. The problem with you is that you think money can make you harmonious, you think relationships can make you harmonious, you think power can make you harmonious, but if your own psyche is not in harmony, nothing can make you harmonious.

Kundalini Yoga works on eight centers, the seven chakras and one engulfing aura. Lots of Kundalini masters have been taught about the chakras. They have not been taught about the arc line and the aura. Therefore, the science is not complete with them. That is why for centuries it has been told that Kundalini Yoga should not be taught because it is dangerous. It is only dangerous if you open up the chakras without the controlling connection of the aura to the arc line. There are ten bodies and they all have to be in balance.

– Yogi Bhajan[32]

Ken Wilber's Integral Map of Consciousness[33] *is a valuable tool to understand how consciousness transcends and includes within you and is the repeated subject of Ken Wilber's Integral Life Theory, which is color-labeled similarly to the chakra system.*

magenta – magical-animistic.
red - egocentric, power, magic-mythic.
amber – mythic, ethnocentric, traditional.
orange – rational, worldcentric, pragmatic, modern
green – pluralistic, multicultural, postmodern
turquoise – global mind, high vision-logic, higher mind
indigo – para-mind, trans-global illumed mind.
violet – mete-mind and overmind

As we have seen, we can't say one of those is right and others wrong; besides, various elements of ALL of those levels are carried forward. As with the holarchy of atoms to molecules to cells to organisms, we wouldn't say, "I want to keep organisms and get rid of atoms and molecules and cells." Likewise, even though we would want to have our worldview informed by as high an altitude as possible, it is not a simple matter of hanging onto violet and jettisoning everything else. - Ken Wilber [33A]

And so it goes with the chakras. If the lower triangle or first, second and third chakras are not developed, then the chakras in the upper triangle cannot be fully actualized. The first chakra is your foundation and supports the potential for each successive level, like building blocks. As a human being, your consciousness was born into the first chakra and as an infant you were egocentric with no awareness of the greater community, other countries, etc. As you continue to develop and grow, your awareness is reflected by your worldview and corresponds to a chakra. Each developmental stage is integrated and included within the next stage. Your highest human potential as an adult is to develop the ability to use your power and individual creativity confidently with compassion and wisdom to engage in peaceful relationships with other individuals, nations, the universe, and beyond.

We all develop at different rates and in different ways. Understanding the chakras helps you to understand yourself and other people. If you can identify from which chakra you are speaking and listening in any situation and from which chakra the person you are speaking to is listening and speaking, true communication can begin to take place.

CHAKRAS[31]

Lower Triangle

First Chakra: Root Chakra, *Muladhara,* red
    Perineum
    Glands: adrenals and testicles
    Earth: *foundations, security, survival, habit, self-acceptance*
    Yoga poses: front stretches, Chair, Crow, lying on the stomach

Second Chakra: *Svadisthana,* orange
    Lower Abdomen
    Glands: ovaries and testicles
    Water, Creativity: *To feel, to desire, to create*
    Yoga poses: Cat-Cow, Sat Kriya, Cobra, Butterfly

Third Chakra: *Manipura,* yellow
- Solar Plexus
- Glands: adrenals and pancreas
- Fire: *action and balance*
- Yoga poses: Stretch Pose, Sat Kriya, Breath of Fire, all exercises for abdominal muscles

Balance Point between Lower and Upper Triangles

Fourth Chakra: *Anahata,* green
- Heart
- Gland: thymus
- Air: *love and compassion*
- Yoga poses: Ego Eradicator, Bear Grip, Child's Pose, Yoga Mudra, all pranayam

Upper Triangle

Fifth Chakra: *Vishudda,* blue
- Throat
- Glands: thyroid and parathyroid
- Sound, Ether: *projective power of the word*
- Yoga Poses: all chanting, Cat-Cow, neck rolls, nose-to-knees

Sixth Chakra: *Ajna,* indigo
- Forehead/Third Eye
- Gland: pituitary
- Light: *intuition, wisdom, identity*
- Yoga Poses: Archer, Yoga Mudra, all exercises where forehead rests on the floor, meditating on the third eye

Seventh Chakra: *Sahasrara*, violet
> Top of head/Crown
> Gland: pineal
> Thought: *humility and vastness*
> Yoga Poses: Ego Eradicator, Sat Kriya, all meditation, concentrating on the tip of the nose

Eighth Chakra: white, all colors, changes with health and state of being.
> The Aura: *radiance*
> *The aura projects the total effects of all the chakras combined.*
> Yoga Poses: Ego Eradicator, Archer, all arm exercises, all meditation

TEN BODIES

Yogi Bhajan taught that you are made up of 10 bodies[34]: 1 physical, 3 mental and 6 energy bodies. The root of all disease exists first in one of the 6 energy bodies before it manifests outwardly. Practicing Kundalini Yoga will strengthen and balance all 10 bodies. Mastering all 10 bodies brings the 11th embodiment or enlightenment, which allows mastery of the physical realm and access to the entire spiritual realm.

The Ten Bodies

1st   Soul Body: *Heart Over Head, Humility, Creativity*
       Key to Balancing: Raise the Kundalini, open the Heart, strengthen first chakra

2nd   Negative Mind: *Longing to Belong, Containment, Obedience*
       Key to Balancing: Value your discipline, develop conscious relationships of integrity, strengthen second chakra

3rd   Positive Mind: *Devil or Divine, Equality, Positivity*
Key to Balancing: Strengthen the navel point, use positive affirmations, strengthen third chakra

4th   Neutral Mind: *Cup of prayer, Service, Compassion, Integration*
Key to Balancing: Meditate, strengthen fourth chakra

5th   Physical Body: *Teacher, Balance, Sacrifice*
Key to balancing: Exercise regularly, teach, strengthen fifth chakra

6th   Arcline: *Person At Prayer, Justice, Protection, Projection*
Arcline extends from earlobe to earlobe across your hairline. It's your halo.
Women have a second arcline extending from nipple to nipple.
Key to Balancing: Awaken the pituitary gland – the third eye, strengthen sixth chakra

7th   Aura: *Platform of Elevation, Mercy, Security, Love*
Electromagnetic field which surrounds your body. It's your shield.
Key to Balancing: Meditate, wear white clothing made of natural fibers, strengthen seventh chakra

8th   Pranic Body: *Finite to infinite, Purity, Energy, Fearlessness, Self-Initiation*
Key to Balancing: All pranayam.

9th   Subtle Body: *Mastery or Mystery, Calmness, Subtlety, Mastery*
Key to Balancing: Do any meditation or kriya for 1,000 days

10th   Radiant Body: *All or Nothing, Royal Courage, Radiance, Nobility*
Key to Balancing: Commitment

11th   Embodiment/Command Center: *Eternal, Flexibility, Completion*
Key to Balancing: Meditative chanting of sacred words

tune in to begin

Always tune in by chanting the Adi Mantra[35] three times.

Adi Mantra means *the first intention expressed as sound.*

The Adi Mantra aligns you to non-dual consciousness, which is you. I-I. It means *I call on the infinite creative consciousness. I call on the subtle consciousness or wisdom within, which brings me from darkness to light.*

Chanting this mantra connects you with the *Golden Chain of Teachers*. The Golden Chain of Teachers is non-dual consciousness. The Divine **I** connects to the Divine **Thou** within the inexpressible Divine **It**. You can listen to it on the Kundalini Research Institute website **www.kriteachings.org** under *Tools for Students and Teachers*.

Ong Namo Guru Dev Namo
Ong Namo Guru Dev Namo
Ong Namo Guru Dev Namo

When you tune in and practice Kundalini Yoga and meditation, you will experience present moment awareness. Present moment awareness is stillness that is always there beneath the surface of busy life, which pulls our focus away from stillness. When you access stillness, it is always the same stillness. It does not change. And your stillness and my stillness are not different. Your personality and thoughts do not affect stillness. As a Yoga teacher, I witness this in class each time. At the point in our meditation where everyone reaches stillness, it is the same stillness for everybody. It's the same for each individual person each time and it's the same stillness for every person in the room at the same time. It's what Eckhart Tolle means by *Now*. It's not Robert's experience of stillness or Heather's experience of stillness. It is stillness, period, unchanged and constantly present. It never changes, it is always, always, always 100% of the time present and it's the same for all of us. Everyone. Always.

Always Now.

Chant

Sit with a straight spine. Place your hands at the heart center in Prayer Pose. With eyes closed, focus at the brow point. Inhale deeply through your nose. Chant:

Ong . . . . . Namo . . . . . Gu-roo Dev . . . . . Na-mo . . . .
.

Chant with one breath, if you are able; otherwise, take a sip of air through the mouth after *Ong Namo*. This chant is done in a monotone with the sound of *Dev* (rhymes with *gave*) a minor third higher than the other sounds. Chant *Ong* so that you feel a vibration at the top of your nose and in the sinuses. Hear the sound and vibrate it within your skull. Repeat three or more times before you practice Kundalini Yoga.

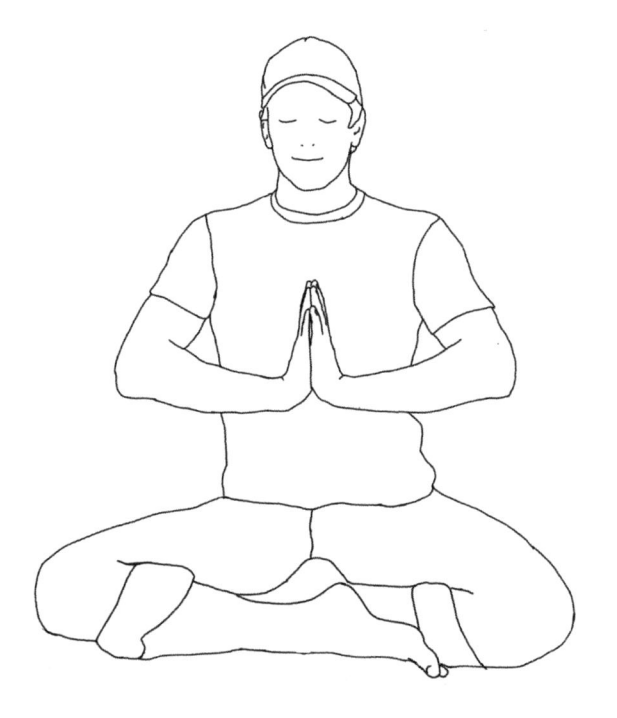

The Complete Adi Mantra for Individual Meditation

Use this mantra as a personal link to connect with the Infinite[36]. The complete individual form of the mantra immerses you in awareness and guidance for your personal situation. It establishes a guiding beam between you in your immediate state and your higher conciousness, which is true through all states.

Ong Namo Guru Dev Namo Guru Dev Namo Guru Dev-a

Sit in Easy Pose with a slight Neck Lock. Focus your eyes at the tip of your nose. Bring both palms in front of the Heart Center facing upward. Touch the sides of your palms along the little fingers and sides of your hands, as if you will receive something in them. Form Gyan Mudra with each hand (page 30).

Chant the entire mantra three to five times on one breath. Keep the number of repetitions per breath constant. The sound *Dayv* is chanted a minor third higher than the other sounds. The sound of *Dayvaa* carries slightly on the *AA* sound.

The sound *ONG* is created in the inner chambers of the sinuses and upper palate. It is the *NG* sound that is emphasized. The first part of *NAMO* is short and rhymes with *HUM*. The syllable *GU* is pronounced as in the word *good*. The syllable *ROO* rhymes with the word *true*. The word *DAYV* rhymes with *save*. The *AA* in *DAYVAA* is chanted with the mouth open and the sound vibrating from an open throat.

Chant for 11-31 minutes for a powerful meditation and guidance. Yogi Bhajan did not restrict longer periods.

It is my experience that by meditating, I enter stillness, I-I and become present to the Now, which is absolute protection from egoic suffering.

practice for present moment awareness[37]

With each exercise, unless otherwise stated, silently hear SAT on your inhale and *NAM* on your exhale. This is an important part of Kundalini Yoga technology because using the mantra powerfully focuses your mind and will dramatically increase your results to bring you to present moment awareness.

With each exercise, unless otherwise stated, lead with your breath. Feel and experience your breath initiating and supporting the movement of the exercise. This brings your practice into the Now.

Unless otherwise stated, an exercise is concluded by inhaling and holding your breath briefly. While the breath is being held, apply the Mulbandha or Root Lock , contracting the muscles around the sphincter, the sex organs and the navel point. Then exhale and relax to allow your body to integrate the effects of the kriya. This consolidates the effect of any exercise and circulates the energy to your higher centers. Do not hold your breath to the point of dizziness. If you start to feel dizzy or faint, immediately exhale and relax.

At the end of each kriya, rest in Corpse Pose for five or more minutes or as directed. Resting allows your system to integrate the positive effects of Yoga, allowing your body to save all the work you've done to boost your immune system, re-align your nervous system and strengthen integration of your body, mind and spirit. This brings peace.

to end

Singing *Longtime Sunshine* and then chanting *Sat Nam* concludes your practice[38].

Singing this song is a prayer of goodwill for all beings. Chanting *Sat Nam* reminds you to hold present moment awareness as you experience your day.

To listen to this closing prayer go to **www.kriteachings.com**. Sing from your heart:

> May the long time sun shine upon you,
> all love surround you
> and the pure light within you guide your way on.

Sat is the true essence of the *all* and *Nam* is that essence in manifestation. As *Sat Nam*, move off the mat and into the world as parent, educator, business mover-and-shaker, athlete, employee, carpenter, administrator, healer, politician, writer, nurse, student, public servant, Yogi, artist, poet, and lover. Perform as many of these services as you like, but do it as your true identity, as the witnessing presence beyond thinking, beyond form, as peace.

> Saaaaaaaaaaaaaaaaaaaaaaaaaaaaaaat Nam

Chant in a monotone. *Sat* rhymes with *what* and *Nam* rhymes with *mom*.

always

All life is Yoga.[39]   – Sri Aurobindo

Surrender through your heart to the Divine Heart that is the creator of all of life.

It's the 21st Century; the Information Age is here, now, and Yoga is accessible to everyone. Cultural beliefs in the past rooted in hierarchical caste systems denied Yoga technology and the resulting experience to most people.

Yoga has always been accessible in the sense that all of the parts of Yoga are naturally occurring processes that are happening to everyone, always. These naturally occurring processes are breathing, moving and vocalizing. Combining and harnessing what comes most naturally to us into a system that we practice and experience accelerates our awareness. This is Yoga technology.

By harnessing the power of conscious breathing, conscious moving and conscious speaking, Witness Consciousness or Divine Shakti is experienced. As Sri Aurobindo noted, we experience *out of normal functions, powers and results, which were always latent but which her ordinary movements do not easily or do not often manifest.*[39A]

Warm-Ups

Yogi Bhajan when leading Kundalini Yoga kriyas, usually did not use warm-ups, although he acknowledged that in some instances warm-ups are useful. Here are some options to choose from if you decide to include a warm-up before practicing a Kundalini Yoga kriya:

- Pranayam sequences are especially good for waking up the body and opening the lungs.

- Do a few repetitions of the short version of Sun Salutations (Surya Namaskara) included in the warm-up section of this book.

- You may choose to practice Spinal Flex, Cat-Cow and Life Nerve Stretches, all of which can stand alone or can be used as a warm-up series. All of these are included in the warm-up section.

SUN SALUTATIONS

When Yogi Bhajan was studying with his teacher, the Sun Salutation was used as a warm-up exercise before starting Kundalini Yoga kriyas. This is an excellent warm-up and is beneficial as an exercise in its own right. It increases cardiac activity and circulation, stretches and bends the spine, massages the inner organs, aids the digestive system, exercises the lungs, and oxygenates the blood.

Synchronize your breath with the movements to create an uninterrupted rhythm throughout the sequence of positions. Start by practicing three rounds and then gradually increase to five or six. When practiced with awareness, this improves one's ability to maximize performance and enjoyment of all Yoga postures.

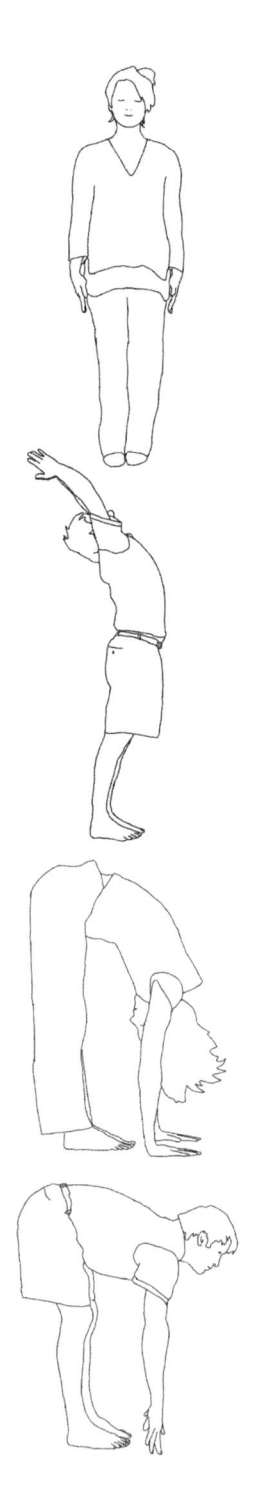

1. **Standing Straight** (Samasthiti)
   Stand up straight, feet together, toes and heels touching, weight evenly distributed between both feet. Find your balance. The arms are by your sides, fingers together.

2. **Stretching Up**
   Inhale, bring your arms up over your head, palms touching. Elongate the spine, lifting the chest and relaxing your shoulders. Be sure not to compress the vertebrae of the neck and lower back. Look up at the thumbs.

3. **Front Bend** (Uttanasana)
   Exhale and bend your torso forward. As you bend forward, keep your spine straight, elongating it as if reaching with the top of the head. When the spine can no longer be held straight, relax the head as close to the knees as possible. Ideally, the chin will be brought to the shins. Keep knees straight and place hands on the floor on either side of the feet, with fingertips and tips of the toes in line. Gaze at the tip of the nose.

4. Inhale, raise the head up, straighten the spine, keeping the hands or fingertips on the floor. Gaze at the Third Eye Point.

5. **Push-up** (Chaturanga Dandasana)
   Exhale and bend the knees, stepping or jumping back so that the legs are straight out behind, balancing on the bottoms of the bent toes. Elbows are bent, hugging the rib cage, and palms are flat on the floor under the shoulders, with fingers spread wide apart. The body is in a straight line from forehead to ankles. Keep yourself equally balanced between hands and feet. Do not push forward with the toes.

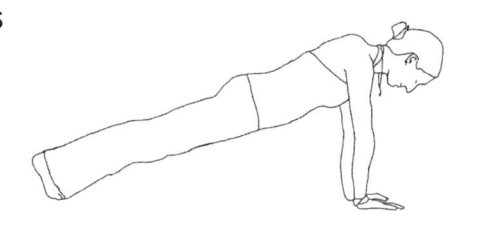

   Author's modification: You may need to lower your knees to help hold your weight in the beginning. Keep your elbows hugging your rib cage and smoothly lower yourself down. Use the navel to keep your lower spine from collapsing.

6. **Cobra Pose** (Bujangasana)
   From this position, inhale, straighten the elbows and arch the back. Stretch through the upper back so that there is no pressure on the lower spine. Point the forehead at the sky and gaze at the tip of the nose. Fingers are spread wide apart.

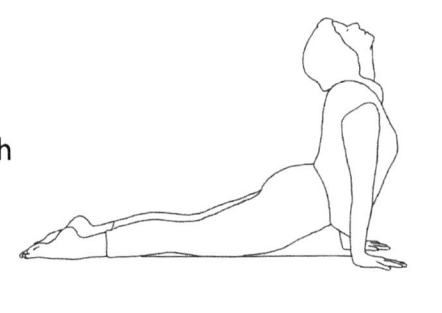

7. **Triangle Pose** (Adho Mukha Svanasana) (AKA Downward Dog)
   Exhale, lift the hips up so that the body is balanced in an inverted v-shape. Feet and palms are flat on the floor, elbows and knees straight. Fingers are spread wide. Gaze toward the navel and hold this position for five breaths.

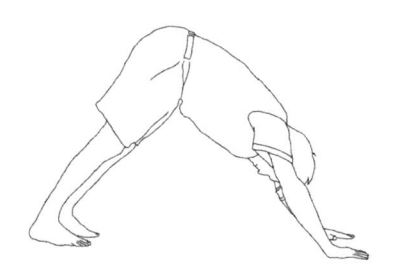

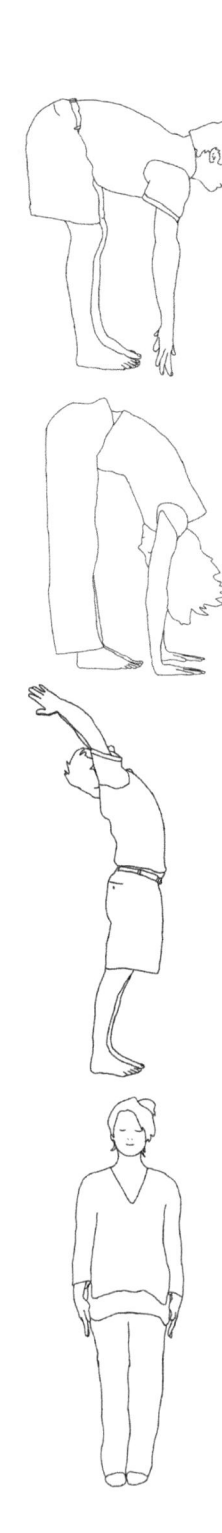

8. Inhale and jump or step back into position #4.

9. **Forward Bend** (Uttanasana)
   Exhale and bend forward into position #3.

10. **Stretching Up**
    Inhale and come all the way up into position #2.

11. **Standing Up** (Samasthiti)
    Exhale and return to the starting position with arms by the sides.

Author's note: I love Sun Salutations because they provide an easy flow and rhythm that allow you to learn to let the breath lead your movement. Before each posture for the Sun Salutation, let the breath lead the movement. This kriya is an example of how to lead with the breath and it applies to each posture in all warm-ups and kriyas, always.

SPINAL SERIES

You can do some or all of these spinal exercises. Always work from the base of the spine up. Spinal twist #3 adjusts and loosens the entire spine. Shoulder shrugs and neck rolls complete the process, allowing spinal fluid to move into the higher centers of your brain, for increased mental clarity and enhanced memory function.

1. **Lower Spinal Flex**
   Sit in Easy Pose. Hold ankles. Inhale, flexing the chest forward and up. Exhale, flexing the spine backwards. Keep your head level, shoulders relaxed. Mentally vibrate *SAT* on the inhale and *NAM* on the exhale. 1-3 minutes

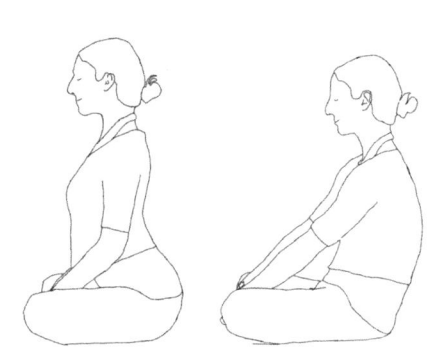

2. **Middle Spinal Flex**
   Sit on your heels with hands flat on thighs. Same breathing and flexing pattern as #1. Mentally vibrate *SAT* on the inhale and *NAM* on the exhale. 1-3 minutes

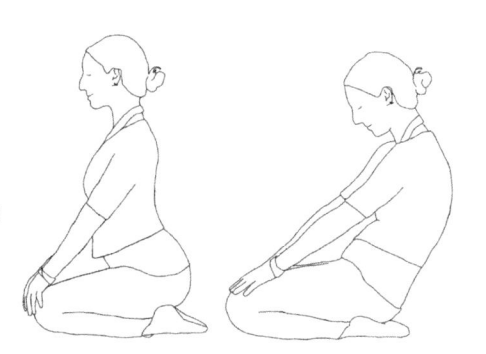

3. **Spinal Twist**
   Sit in Easy Pose. Hold shoulders, fingers in front and thumbs in back. Inhale, twist left, exhale, and twist right. Rotate from the navel point. Head twists with your spine in Neck Lock. Mentally vibrate *SAT* on the inhale and *NAM* on the exhale. 1-3 minutes

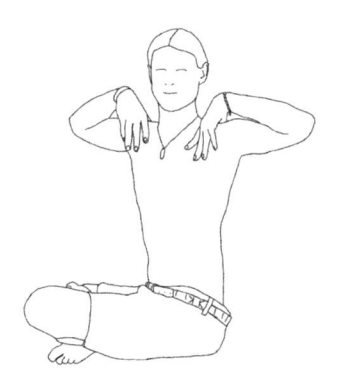

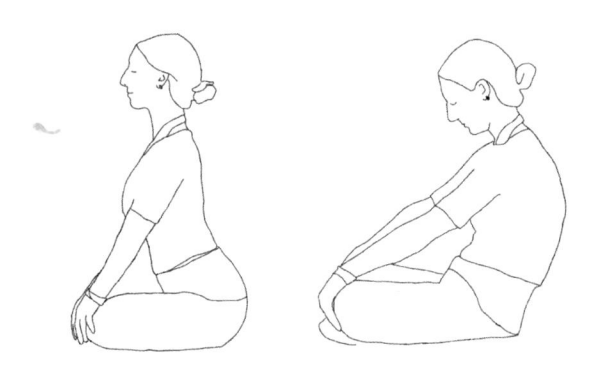

4. **Upper Spinal Flex**
Sit in Easy Pose. Hold knees firmly. Keep elbows straight. Same breathing and flexing pattern as #2. Mentally vibrate *Sat* on the inhale and *Nam* on the exhale. 1-3 minutes

Author's note: Feel a release between the shoulder blades as the heart opens.

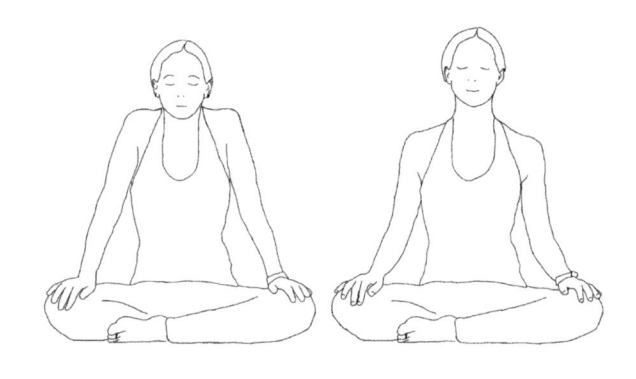

5. **Shoulder Shrugs**
Sit in Easy Pose. Inhale, squeeze shoulders up, exhale, and relax shoulders down. Mentally vibrate *SAT* on the inhale and *NAM* on the exhale. Repeat for less than 2 minutes. Inhale. Hold breath with shoulders up for 15 seconds. Release.

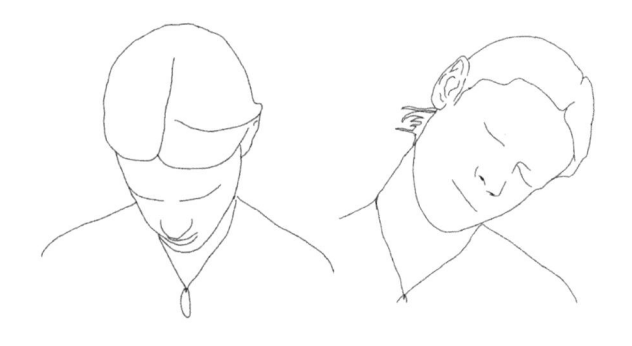

6. **Neck Rolls**
Sit in Easy Pose. Gently bring your chin towards the chest. Slowly rotate the head in a complete oval five times to the right and then five times to the left. Mentally vibrate *SAT* on the inhale and *NAM* on the exhale. Inhale and bring your head back to center. Release.

Author's note: Relax the neck muscles during the exercise.

Life Nerve Stretch (Front Stretch)

Stretching the legs out fully allows you to stretch and strengthen the sciatic nerve. Tension is released in your lower back and legs.

1. Begin by sitting down with the legs stretched out in front. Grab the big toes in finger lock. (Index finger and middle finger pull the toe and the thumb presses the nail of the toe.

2. Exhale, lengthening the spine, bending forward from the navel, continuing to lengthen the spine.

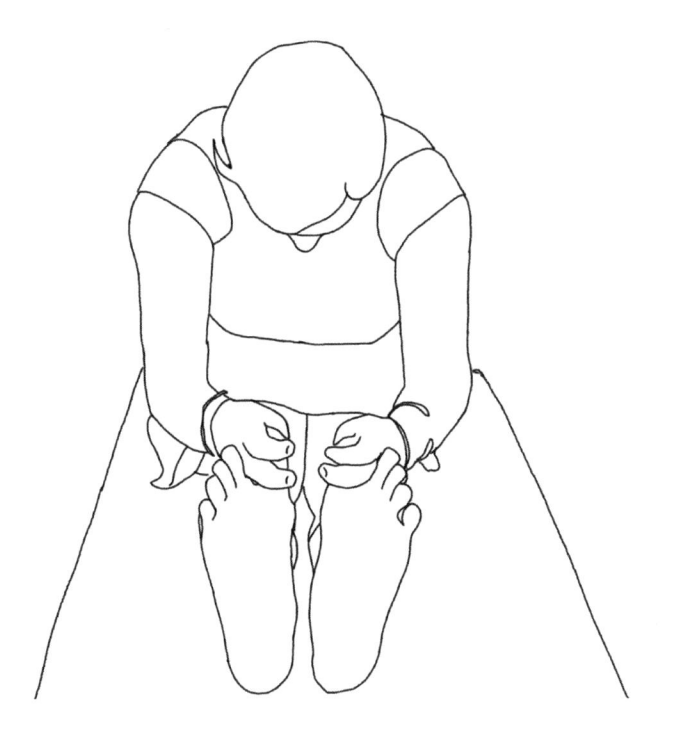

3. Inhale, use the legs to push up. The head follows last. Don't lead with the head. Reverse to come up: head comes up last.

Checkpoints: Lead with the navel point, never with the head. Do not compress the lower back. Try to get the belly to the thighs rather than the head to the knees. Tighten the thigh muscles and pull them away from the knees to hold the stretch.

Author's modification: Take hold of the big toes, ankles or anyplace on your legs that you can reach while keeping your spine as straight as possible and move from there.

Life Nerve Stretch (Left and Right)

1. Begin by sitting down with the legs stretched out in front. Bend the left leg and bring the left heel close to the groin.

2. Grab the right big toe in finger lock with the fingers of the right hand. Index finger and middle finger pulling the toe and the thumb pressing the nail of the toe. The left hand grabs the sole of the right foot.

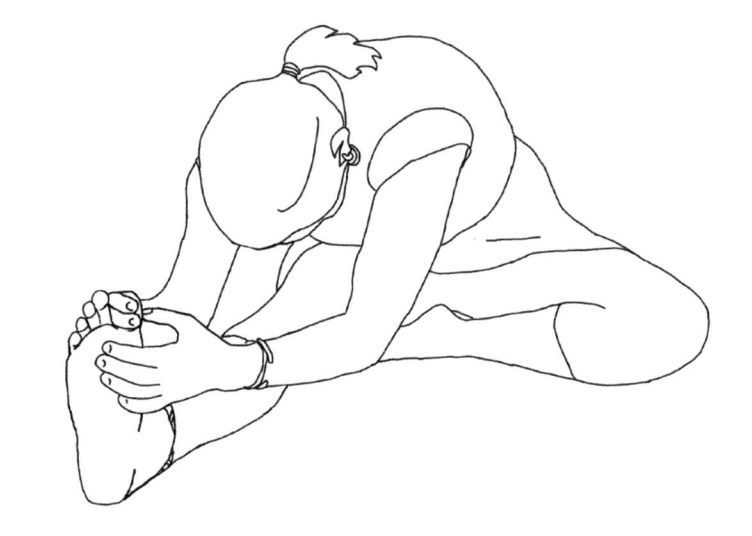

3. Inhale up, turn to your right, lengthen the spine.

4. Exhale, bend forward from the navel, continuing to lengthen the spine. The head follows, last.

5. Reverse to come up: Head comes up last.

6. Do the same on the left side.

Checkpoints: Lead with the navel, never with the head. Pull with the arms to help lengthen the spine on the exhale. Do not compress the lower back. If you can't quite achieve the full stretch, grab the ankle or whatever you can reach.

Cat-Cow

This exercise brings flexibility to your spine, including your cervical vertebrae, and circulates your spinal fluid.

1. Begin on the hands and knees. Hands are shoulder-width apart with fingers facing forward.

2. The knees are directly under the hips.

3. Inhale and tilt the pelvis forward, arching the spine down (Cow position) with head and neck stretched back. Do not scrunch the neck. Open the heart and raise the chin as far back as you can without collapsing the neck.

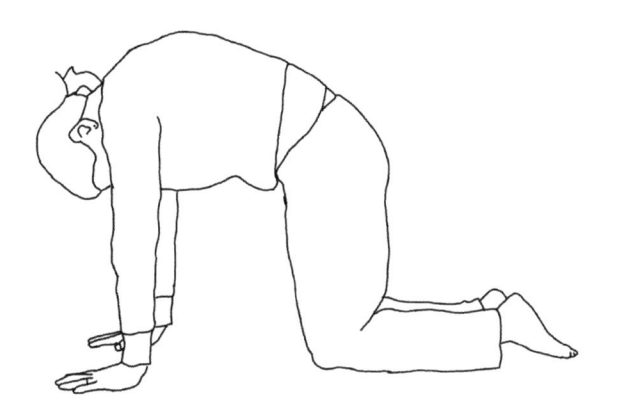

4. Exhale and tilt the pelvis the opposite way, arching the spine up (Cat position), pressing the chin into the chest.

Checkpoints: Keep the motion smooth, moving from the bottom to the top. The head moves last. Start off slowly. Then when the movement is established, you can speed up. *You can go as fast as you want, as long as your head moves last.* Inhale into the extended position and hold a little bit of tension at the navel point. This allows for more widening of the hips.

Author's notes: If this puts a strain on the wrists, you can move the hands forward or rest your weight on closed fists instead of flat palms.

Baby Pose

This posture opens and strengthens your heart muscles. Your heart is elevated higher than your head. Take the opportunity while in this pose to ask yourself what it is that you bow to.

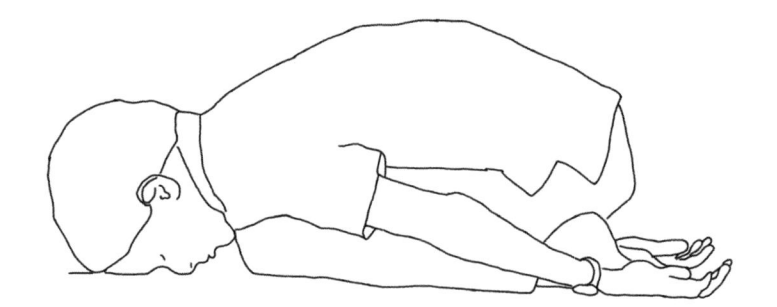

1. Begin by sitting on the heels.

2. Bend forward and place the forehead on the ground, putting pressure on the Third Eye.

3. Arms are at your sides with palms facing up

Author's note: I also teach this variation: Sit on your heels and spread your knees. Bend forward, placing your forehead on the floor. Your arms are stretched out in front of you with fingers spread and palms down.

Author's modification: Place a cushion or rolled up blanket to shorten your distance to the floor.

Archer Pose

This posture strengthens your ability to focus with power and determination. It will help you overcome confusion and vulnerability and increase your power of projection. Physical stamina in your feet, thighs, arms, and intestines is enhanced. This pose puts pressure on your thigh bone, balancing vital minerals: calcium, potassium, magnesium, and sodium.

1. Begin in a standing position.

2. Spread the feet approximately 2-3 feet apart, depending on your size.

3. Place the right foot forward. Place the left foot at right angles to the right foot. Push forward, so that the right knee is over the right toes.

4. Stretch the left leg behind with the knee straight. Tuck the tailbone under using the internal muscles.

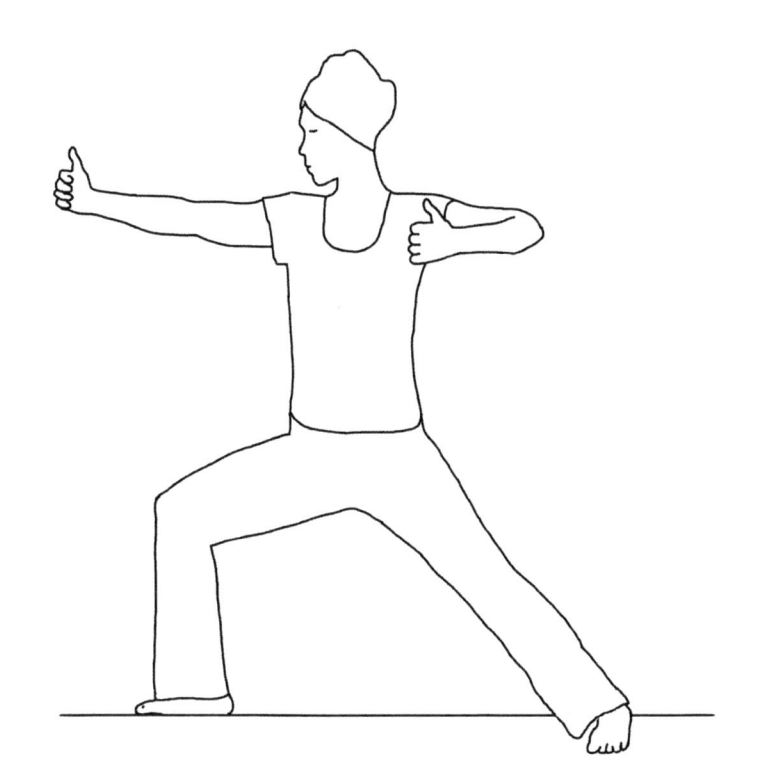

5. Curl the fingers of both hands onto the palms, thumbs pulled back. As if pulling back a bow and arrow, lift the right arm up, extended forward parallel to the ground, over the right knee. The left arm, bent at the elbow, will be "pulling" back.

6. Pull Neck Lock. Chin in. Chest out.

7. Do the same posture on the opposite side.

Checkpoints: Feel the stretch across the hips, just under the hipbones. Avoid over-arching, so there is no sway in the back. Balance the weight on both legs. Keep the back elbow parallel to the ground.

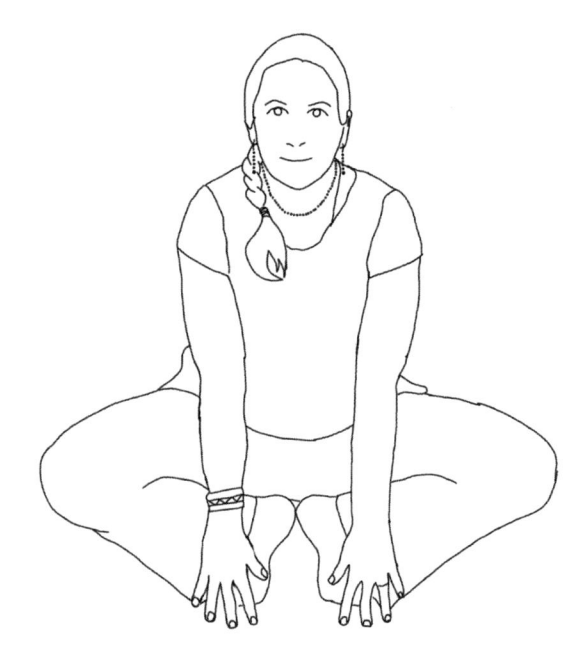

Frog Pose

This exercise powerfully moves internal heat (*tapas*) and energy up the spine, beginning from the lower triangle of chakras (elimination, creativity and will), up through the heart and into the upper triangle of chakras (vocalization, intuition and vastness). Physically, this exercise balances the glandular system.

1. Squat down on the toes. The heels are touching and raised up.

2. Place the fingertips on the ground between the legs.

3. The face is forwards.

4. Inhale as you raise the hips up, keeping the fingertips on the ground, heels up, knees locked.

5. Exhale back; face is forward, knees outside of arms.

6. The movement is rapid.

Author's note: Allow the breath to lead the movement. (I find it helps to feel your inhale lift you up and feel your exhale bring you down.) Repeat for 13-26 repetitions. Gradually increase to 108 maximum repetitions.

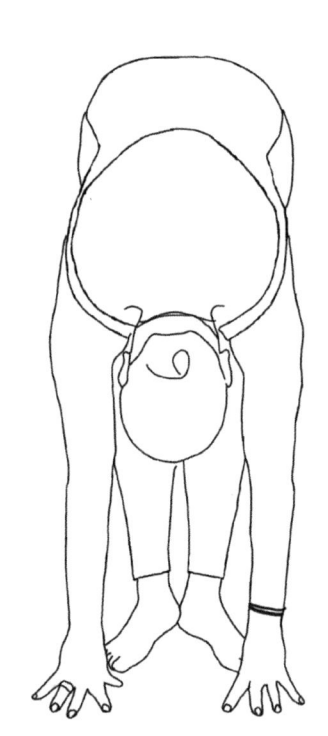

HIP STRETCHES

Butterfly

1. Begin in Easy Pose

2. Grab underneath the feet and hold the soles of the feet together.

3. Pull the spine up.

4. Apply Neck Lock.

5. Bounce the knees, coordinated with the breath.

Butterfly Bend

1. Begin in Easy Pose

2. Grab underneath the feet and hold the soles of the feet together.

3. Pull the spine up.

4. Apply Neck Lock.

5. Bend forward, lengthening the spine. Do not lead with the head, initiate with the navel.

6. As you exhale, draw the navel in and up.

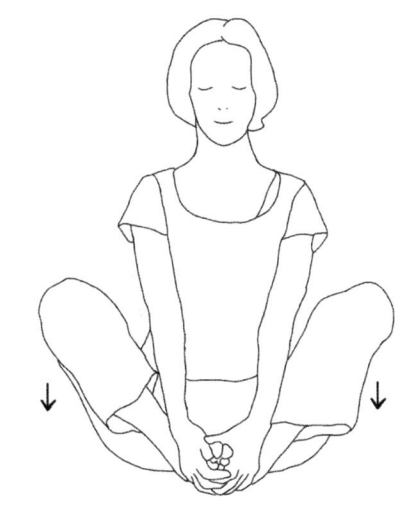

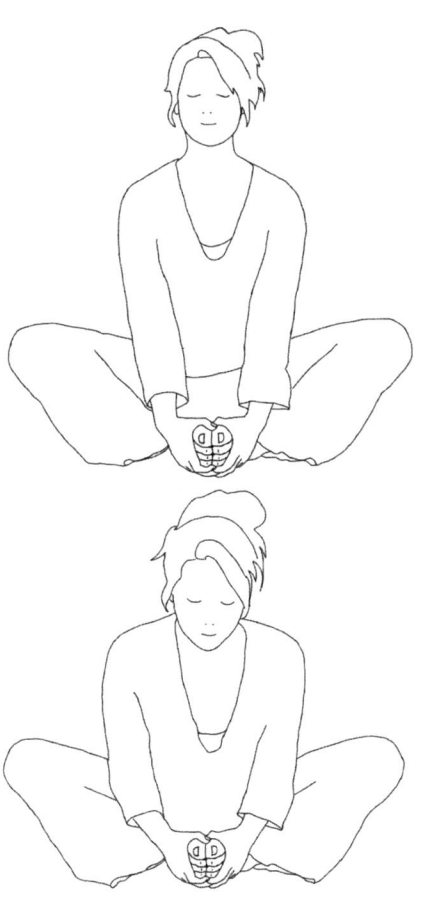

Side Stretch

1. Begin by sitting down with the legs stretched out in front.

2. Bend the left leg and bring the left heel close to the groin.

3. Grab the right big toe in finger lock with the fingers of the right hand. (Index finger and middle finger pulling the toe and the thumb pressing the nail of the toe.)

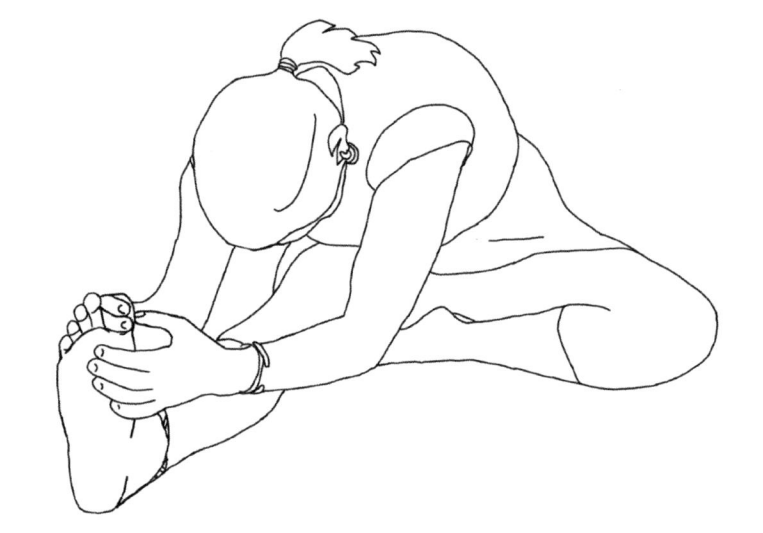

4. The left hand grabs the sole of the right foot.

5. Inhale up, turn to your right, lengthen the spine.

6. Exhale, bend forward from the navel, continuing to lengthen the spine.

7. The head follows, last.

8. Reverse to come up. Head comes up last.

9. Do the same on the left side.

Checkpoints: Lead with the navel, never the head. Pull with the arms to help lengthen the spine on the exhale. Do not compress the lower back. If you can't quite achieve the full stretch, grab the ankle or whatever you can reach.

Triangle (AKA Downward Dog)

1. Begin in a standing position.

2. Place the palms of the hands with the fingers spread wide and the soles of the feet on the ground. The feet are approximately hip-width apart.

3. Create a straight line between your wrists and your hips and from your hips to your heels.

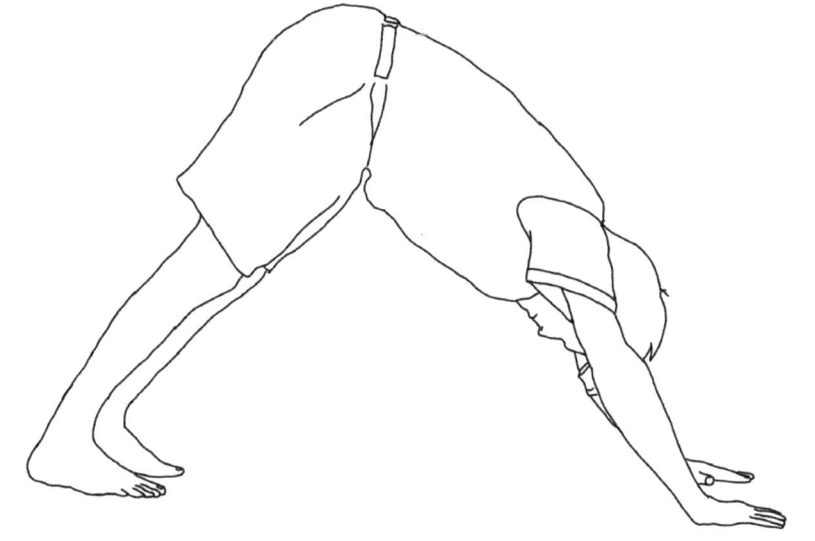

4. The chin is pulled in, elongating the neck.

5. Roll the armpits toward each other.

6. Do not over-sway the back.

ENERGIZING WARM-UP SERIES

Stretch Pose, Nose to Knees Pose and Ego Eradicator

These three exercises are excellent when you first wake up even before you get out of bed. Practice to tap into the eternal flow of energy ready to serve you. Saying *yes* to your practice allows life to start working for you rather than against you. Do each exercise for 30 seconds -3 minutes in the following order.

Stretch Pose

1. Feet are together. Press the lower back into the floor using a pelvic tilt, using the muscles of the navel and *mulbandh*.

2. Put the hands wherever it feels most natural, either palms facing the thighs alongside the body or hands over the thighs, palms down.

3. Lift the head up by lifting the heart up.

4. Apply Neck Lock.

5. Look at the toes.

6. Lift the feet up six inches.

7. Begin Breath of Fire.

Checkpoints: You may use one leg at a time and keep the Breath of Fire powerful.

Nose To Knees Pose

1. Begin by lying on the back.

2. Bend knees and hug them to the chest.

3. Raise the head, bringing the nose towards the knees, between the knees if possible.

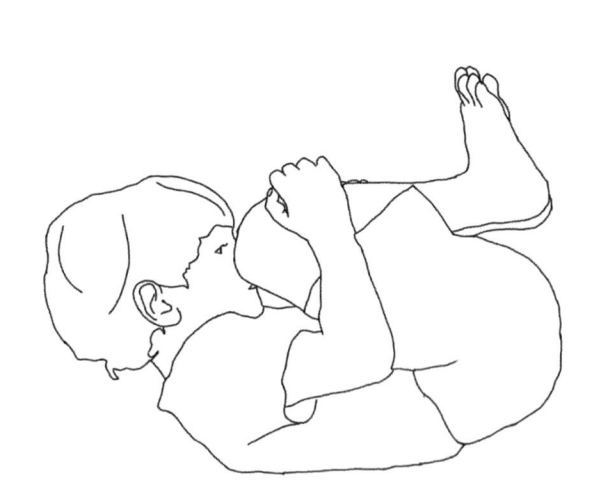

4. Begin Breath of Fire.

Author's modification: Before you begin the exercise, bend your knees to your chest, breathe long and deeply for a few breaths, enjoying the sensation of stretch, and direct the breath through your heart. Make sure to bring your head back to the floor if this exercise causes too much tension in the neck or head.

Ego Eradicator

1. Begin by sitting on the heels or in easy pose.

2. Apply Neck Lock.

3. Lift the arms up 60 degrees. Then draw the shoulder blades down over the back of the ribs so the shoulders are away from the ears.

4. Curl the fingertips onto the pads of the palms with the thumbs stretched back. Create a straight line on the inside of the arm, without a break in the wrist to the tip of the thumbs.

5. To end, touch the thumbs above the head and open fingers.

Checkpoints: Do not bend the elbows. Stretch up from the shoulders. Do not arch the spine and check the angle of the arms.

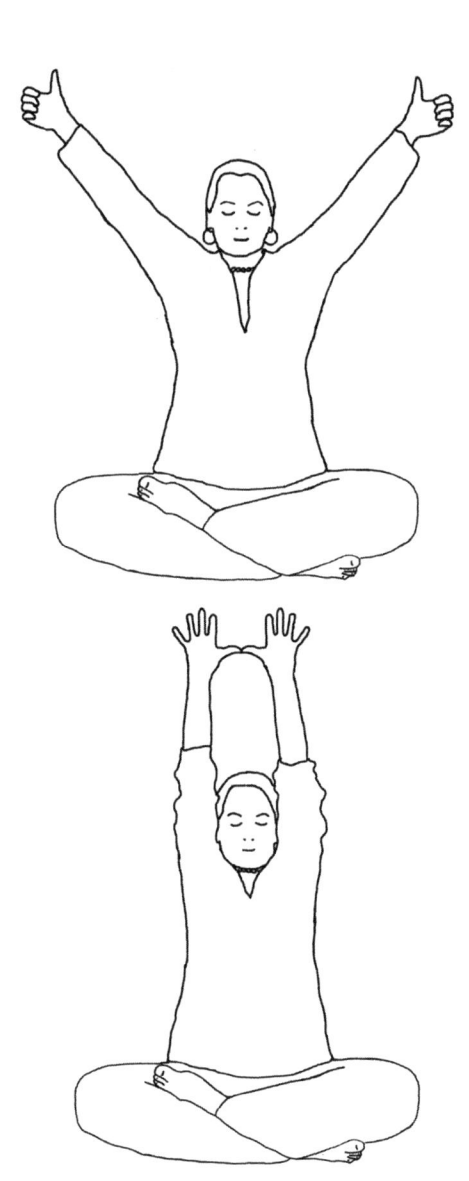

a meditation and kriya for all seasons

Experience and believe.[40] — Yogi Bhajan

Author's note: The Beginner's Meditation and Sat Kriya, practiced regularly, will transform your body, mind and spirit. As you meditate, continue to notice your breath and noticing that you are noticing.

Beginner's Meditation is a simple, effective meditation to do anytime.

Sit in Easy Pose with your eyes closed. Breathe long and deep and follow the flow of your breath. Stay aware of your expanding abdomen on your inhale and notice how it contracts while emptying on the exhale. After a short time, allow your awareness to rest at the heart center and notice your breath. Deepen each breath. Consciously breathe into the heart center, opening and releasing any amount of tension. If you like, you can silently use a mantra with the breath such as *Sat* on the inhale and *Nam* on the exhale.

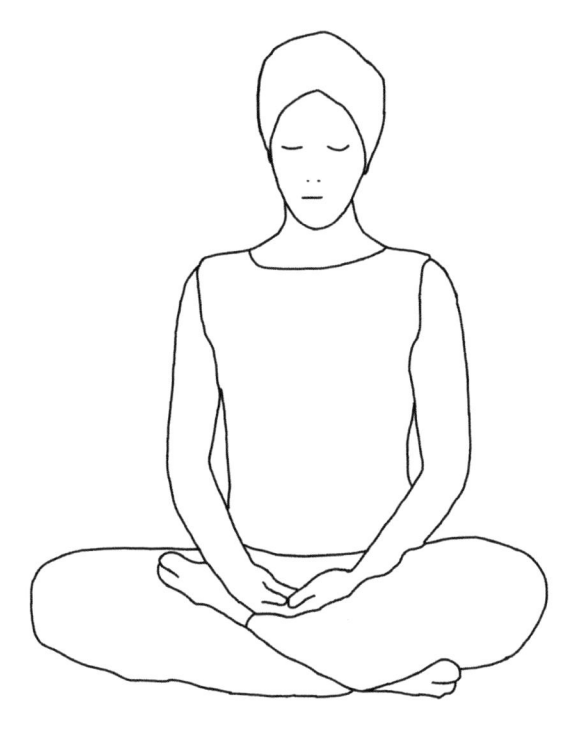

Continue to breathe slowly and deeply as you move your awareness from the heart center to the brow point, also called the Third Eye or Ajna Chakra. Your eyes are still closed and now looking between the eyebrows and inward a little bit. This gaze at the Third Eye puts pressure on your pituitary gland, stimulating it to secrete hormones that enhance intuition and stimulate your immune system. Continue to notice the flow of your breath, and after another minute or so, move your attention back to the heart center. Notice how each focal point makes you feel.

As you continue to breathe deeply, hold your attention at your heart center and your third eye at the same time. Notice how this feels. There should be no strain. Continue *playing* with this meditation for as long as you like. When you are finished, inhale deeply and stretch your spine up and your arms overhead, shaking them vigorously for 10 seconds or so. Relax.

Sat Kriya, practiced for at least three minutes every day, was recommended by Yogi Bhajan. Sat Kriya must be experienced to believe its powerful effect. Use it in place of, or in addition to, any other kriya in your daily practice when practiced for 11 minutes or longer. Regular practice will generate tremendous healing energy, stimulate circulation, increase lung capacity, raise energy up your spine to combine passion with compassion, strengthen your entire sexual system, strengthen your heart, regulate blood pressure, and improve your over-all health. Begin practicing for 3 minutes and slowly build over time. This is a very powerful exercise, so respect the power of this technique and build gradually. A compassionate way to increase your time is to practice for 3 minutes and then rest for 2. Repeat this cycle, gradually adding cycles until you have completed 15 minutes of Sat Kriya and 10 minutes of rest. Completing 31 minutes of Sat Kriya is an advanced practice. Keep it real!

Reminder: If you have high blood pressure, please consult your physician before practicing this or any other Yoga meditation or kriya.

How to Do Sat Kriya

- Sit on the heels with the arms overhead and palms together. Interlace the fingers except for the index fingers, which point straight up. Men cross the right thumb over the left thumb; women cross the left thumb over the right.

- Chant SAT and pull the navel point in; chant NAAM and relax it. Chant with a constant rhythm of about 8 times per 10 seconds. As you pull the navel in and up towards the spine, chant (sucking in the sound) SUT from the navel point. Feel the pressure from the Third Chakra center. With the sound NAAM , relax the belly. The focus of the sound NAAM can be either at the Navel Point or at the Brow Point.

- The breath regulates itself. No breath focus is necessary.

- The spine stays still and straight. The rhythmic contraction and relaxation produces waves of energy that circulate, energize and heal the body. This is neither a spinal flex nor a pelvic thrust. Remain firmly seated on the heels throughout the motions of the kriya.

To end: Inhale, apply Root Lock *(Mulbandh)* and squeeze the muscles tightly from the buttocks all the way up the back, along the spine, past the shoulders. Mentally allow the energy to flow through the top of the skull. Exhale, hold the breath out and apply all the locks *(Mahabandh)*. Inhale and relax. If you practice this as a complete kriya in itself, the relaxation is ideally twice the length of time as you practiced the Sat Kriya. (If practiced as part of a kriya, follow the relaxation times specified.)

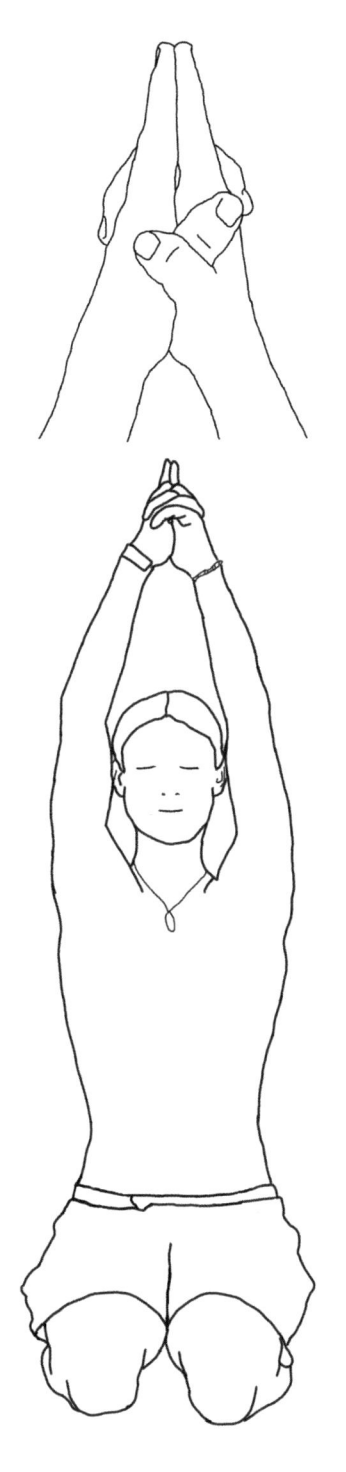

spring equinox

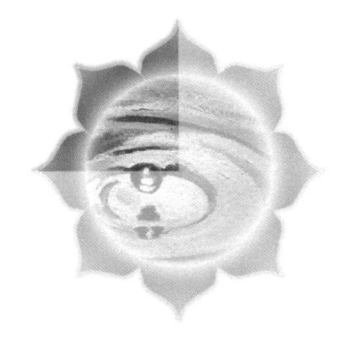

Reminders
- *Tune in to begin (page 53).*
- *Use the Neck Lock (page 16) in all postures unless otherwise stated.*
- *Unless otherwise stated, the mantra **Sat Nam** can be used during all exercises with each breath by silently vibrating Sat on the inhale and Nam on the exhale. End each exercise by inhaling deeply and applying the Root Lock (page 15) with the breath held in for 5- 15 seconds. Exhale.*
- *Close your session by singing **Longtime Sunshine** and chanting one long **Sat Nam**.*

KRIYA

Basic Spinal Energizer Series

Age is measured by the flexibility of the spine: To stay young, stay flexible. This series works systematically from the base of the spine to the top. All 26 vertebrae receive stimulation and all the chakras receive a burst of energy. This makes it a good series to do before meditation. Many people report greater mental clarity after regular practice of this kriya. A contributing

---

Air, spring, yellow, the mind, intellect, power of thought to shape your world, East, a time of new life, germination, overcoming winter and death, light and warmth increases.

Air is the inspiration of life-giving breath. Air is the power of sound as vocalization of ideas and the communication of knowledge.

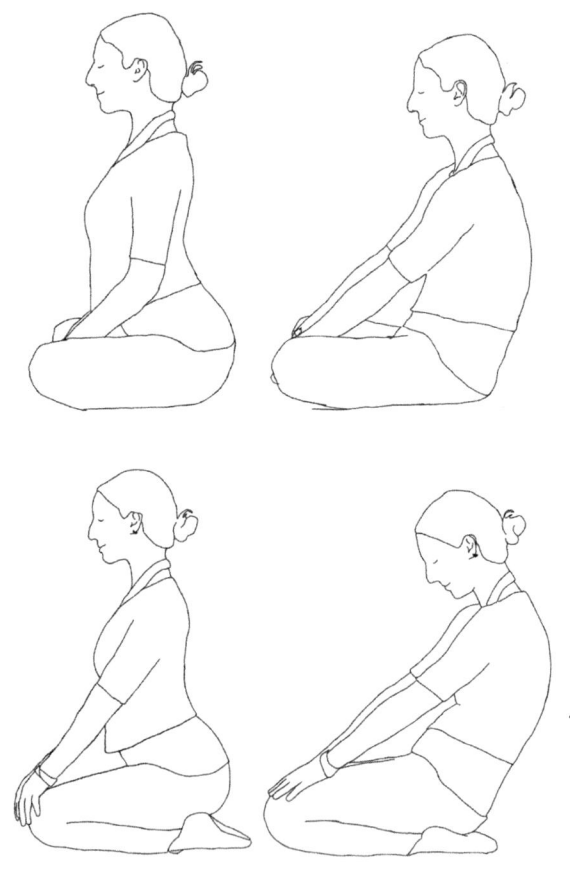

factor is the increased circulation of the spinal fluid, which is crucially linked to having a good memory.

1. **Spinal Flex**
   Sit in Easy Pose. Grab the ankles with both hands and deeply inhale. Flex the spine forward and lift the chest up. On the exhale, flex the spine backwards. Keep the head level so it does not *flip-flop*. Repeat 108 times. Rest 1 minute. Spinal flexes have a "multi-stage reaction pattern" that greatly alters the proportions and strengths of alpha, theta and delta waves.

2. **Spinal Flex**
   Sit on the heels. Place the hands flat on the thighs. Flex spine forward on the inhale, backward on the exhale. Mentally vibrate *Sat* on the inhale, and *Nam* on the exhale. Repeat up to 108 times. Rest 2 minutes.

3. **Spinal Twist**
   In Easy Pose, grasp the shoulders with fingers in front, thumbs in back. Inhale and twist to the left, exhale and twist to the right. Breathing is long and deep. Continue 26 times and inhale facing forward. Rest 1 minute.

4. **Bear Grip**

   Lock your fingers in Bear Grip at the heart center. Clasping hands, your left palm faces out from chest, thumb on the bottom. Right palm faces chest with thumb on the top. Curl the fingers of both hands so they form a fist. Move your elbows in a seesaw motion, breathing long and deeply in rhythm with the movement. Continue 26 times and inhale, exhale, pull Root Lock. Relax 30 seconds.

5. **Spinal Flex**

   In Easy Pose, grasp the knees firmly. Keeping your elbows straight, begin to flex the upper spine. Inhale forward, exhale back. Repeat 108 times. Rest 1 minute.

6. **Shoulder Shrugs**

   Shrug both shoulders up on the inhale and down on the exhale. Do this for less than 2 minutes. Inhale and hold 15 seconds with shoulders pressed up. Relax the shoulders.

7. **Neck Rolls**

   Roll the neck slowly to the right five times, then to the left five times. Inhale and pull the neck straight.

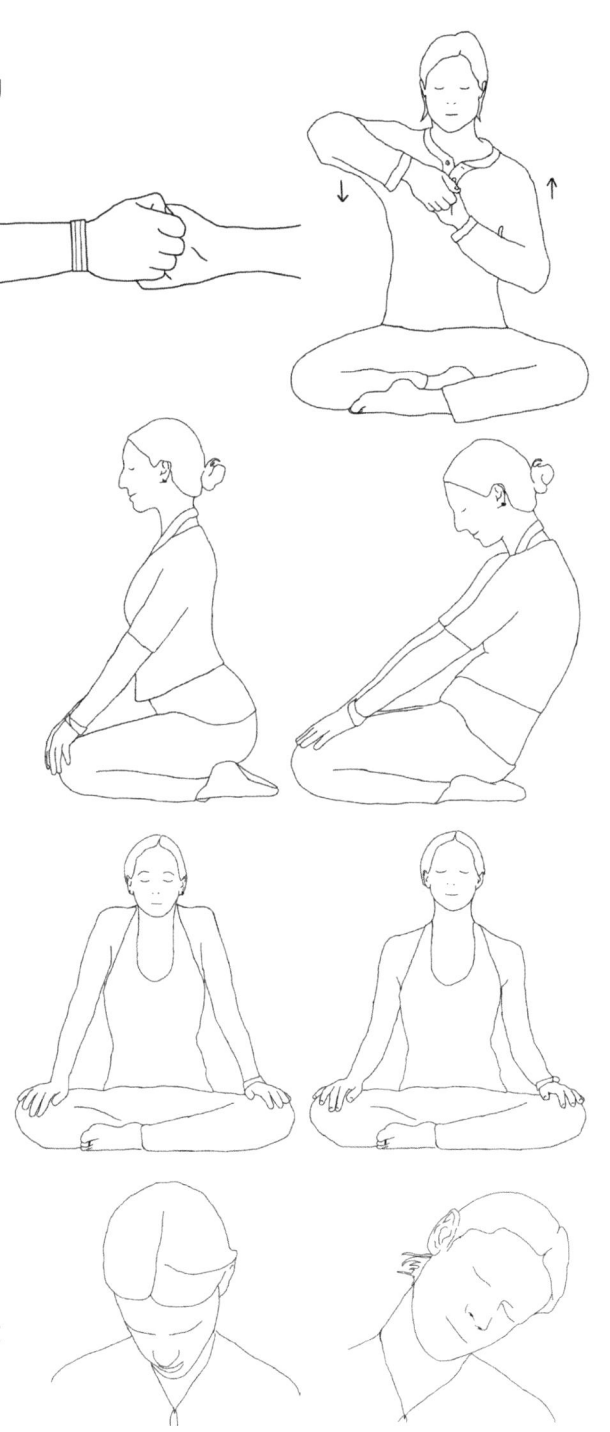

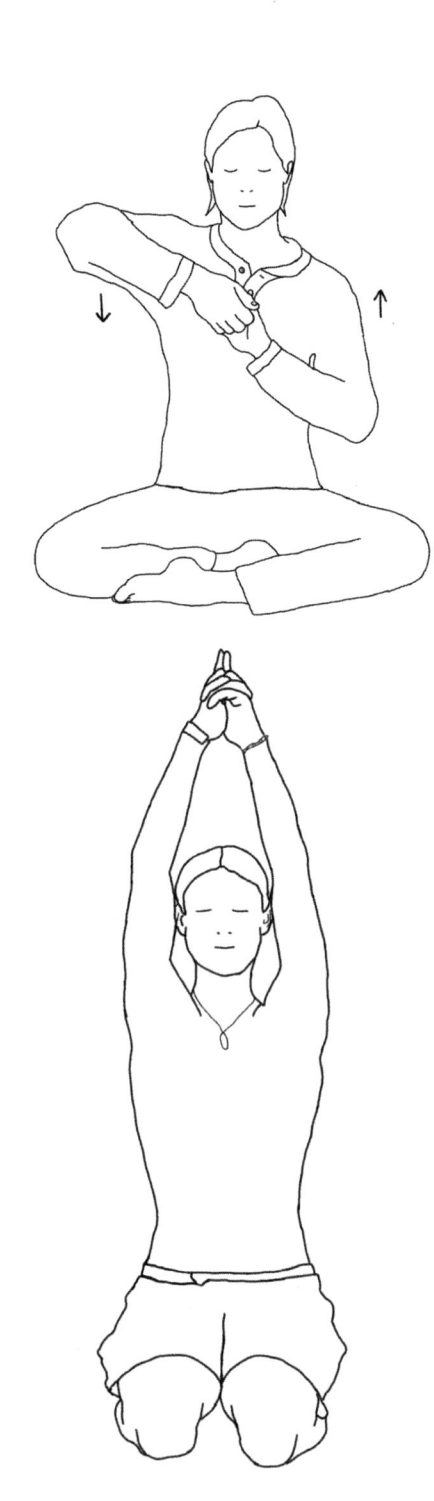

8. **Bear Grip**

   Lock the fingers in Bear Grip at the throat level. Inhale and apply Mulbandh. Exhale and apply Mulbandh. Then raise the hands above the top of the head. Inhale and apply Mulbandh. Exhale and apply Mulbandh. Repeat the cycle 2 more times.

9. **Sat Kriya**

   Sit on heels with the arms overhead and the palms together. Interlace the fingers except for the index fingers, which point straight up. Men cross the right thumb over the left thumb; women cross the left thumb over the right. Chant *Sat* and pull the Navel Point in, chant *Naam* and relax it. Continue powerfully with a steady rhythm for at least 3 minutes, then inhale, apply Root Lock and squeeze the energy from the base of the spine to the top of the skull. Exhale, hold the breath out and apply all the locks. Inhale and relax.

Checkpoints: Beginners, each exercise that lists 108 repetitions can be done 24 times. The rest periods are then extended from 1 to 2 minutes.

KRIYA

Wahe Guru Kriya | Originally taught November 27, 1974.

You have to experience this kriya to know its tremendous benefit. It will make you sweat and is a total workout for the thyroid, pituitary and pineal glands.

1. Come into *Chair Pose* (knees bent, back parallel to the ground, hands resting flat on tops of the feet.) *[Author's modification*: If that is not possible, I instruct students to grasp their heels.] Keep the spine straight. The head faces down. Turn the head to the left and say WHA-HAY. Turn the head to the right and say GUROO. Alternate at a moderate pace to make a continuous sound current. WHA-HAY GUROO, WHA-HAY GUROO, WHA-HAY GUROO. Continue for three minutes.

2. Stand up straight. Put hands on the hips and lean backwards. Keep the legs straight. Let the head fall back. Turn head to the left and say WHA-HAY. Turn head to the right and say GUROO. Continue for three minutes.

3. Stand up straight. Bend slightly so the hands rest on the knees. Spine is straight but head is up. Chant WHA-HAY while turning the head to the left. Chant GUROO while turning the head to the right. Continue for three minutes.

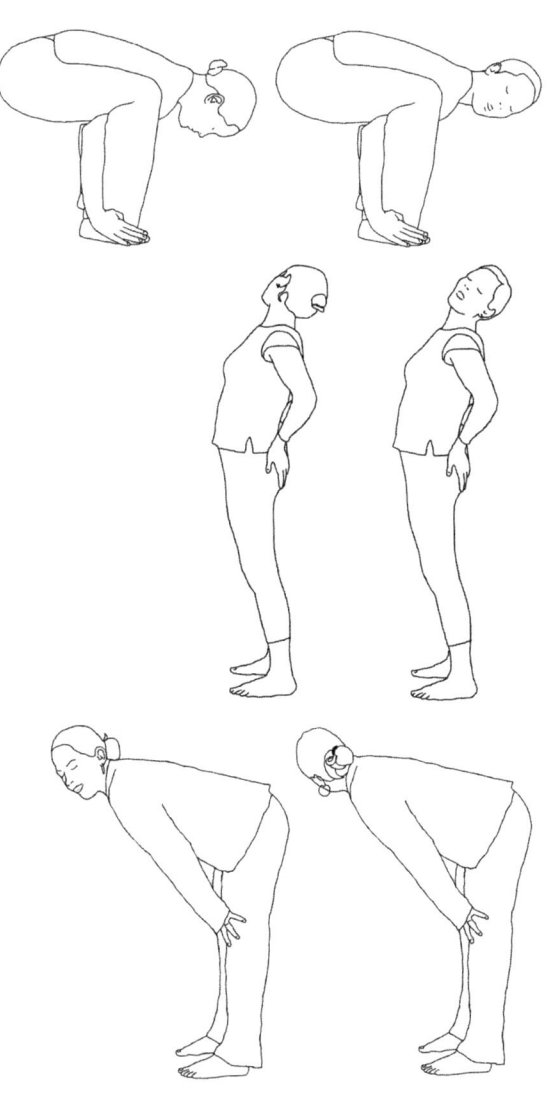

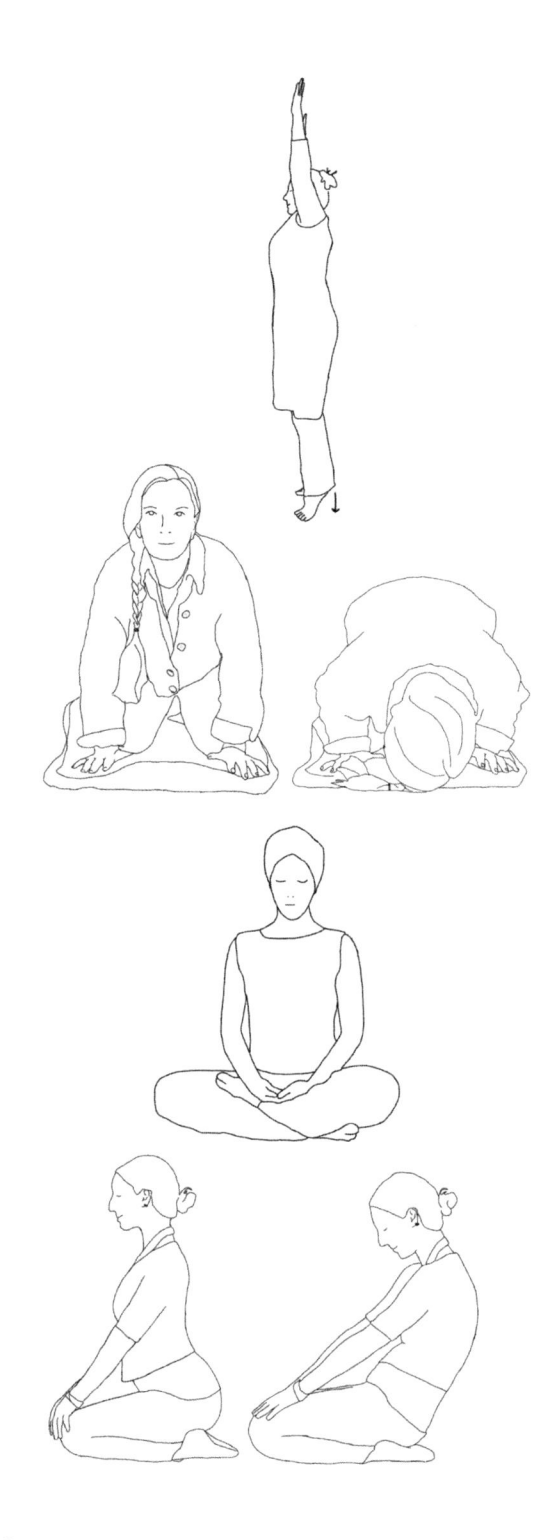

4. *Stand Up Stretch* - Stand up. Stretch arms straight overhead. On WHA-HAY, the feet are flat on the ground. With GUROO, rise up on the toes. Continue for three minutes

5. *Sphinx.* Sit on heels. Place the palms flat on the floor just in front of the knees. Spine and arms are straight looking like a sphinx. Bend forward, touching the forehead to the ground and chant GUROO. Rise up and chant WHA-HAY. Continue for three minutes.

6. Sit in *Easy Pose*. Begin to whisper the Panj Shabd: SAA-TAA-NAA-MAA. After two minutes, chant loudly for two more minutes.

7. *Spinal Flex With Chanting* — Immediately come onto the heels with palms on the thighs. Begin flexing the spine, and with a powerful whisper, chant *SAA* forward, *TAA* back, *NAA* forward, *MAA* back. Continue for three minutes, then meditate.

Checkpoints: While chanting WHA, focus at the navel point. With HAY, focus at the chest and with GUROO, focus on the pursed lips. Teaching this kriya, I instruct my students to focus on the sound of their voice as they chant the mantra and to stay with the sound.

Meditation

Fight Brain Fatigue | Originally taught March 27, 1995.

This exercise fights brain fatigue and balances your diaphragm. You will renew blood supply to your brain and move serum in your spine. It will also benefit your lymphatic system, liver, spleen, and navel point.

1. Sit in Easy Pose with your elbows bent and your upper arms near your rib cage. Your forearms point straight out in front of your body, parallel to the floor. The right palm faces downward and the left palm faces upward. Breathing through your nose, inhale in eight strokes. On each stroke of the breath, alternately move your hands up and down. One hand moves up as the other hand moves down. The movement of the hands is slight, approximately six to eight inches. Then change hand position so that the left palm faces downward and the right palm faces upward. Continue for another three minutes and then change the hand position again so that the right palm faces downward and the left palm faces upward. Continue for a final three minutes (Total time for this part of the meditation is nine minutes).

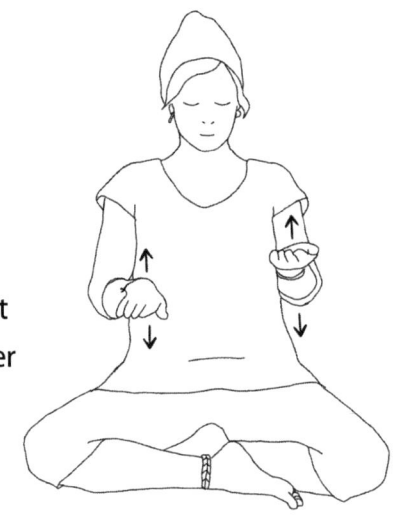

2. Begin long, slow, deep breathing, stopping the movement and holding the position. Close your eyes and focus at the center of your chin. Keep your body perfectly still so it can heal itself. Keep your mind quiet, stilling your thoughts. 5 ½ minutes.

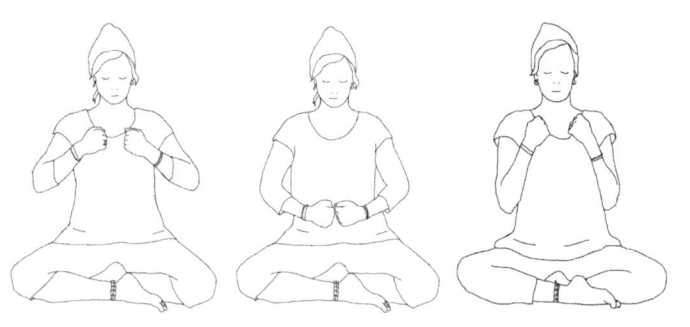

To finish: Inhale deeply, hold your breath, make your hands into fists, and press them strongly against your chest. 15 seconds. Exhale. Inhale deeply, hold your breath and press your fists against your navel point. 15 seconds. Exhale. Inhale deeply, hold your breath, bend your elbows, bringing your fists near your shoulders, and press your arms strongly against your rib cage. 15 seconds. Exhale and relax.

Chanting Meditation

The Divine Shield Meditation For Protection and Positivity | Originally taught in September 1971.

It is nearly impossible to solve the problems that upset you. When your aura is weak, it extends out from your body less than four feet and you tend to become depressed and cannot fight off negativity coming from within or from the environment. By practicing this meditation, you temporarily extend your aura out (up to nine feet in all directions). The outer aura acts as a filter and connector to the universal magnetic field. The compassion of the universe uplifts and expands you as you chant *MA* to activate and open the heart center. You will feel yourself move in rhythm with your true identity as part of the greater reality. With regular practice, your shield becomes strong and you will be positive, fearless and happy, protected even from the impact of your past actions.

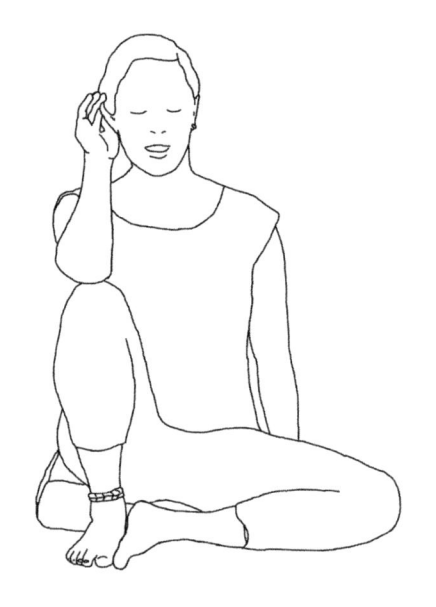

Posture – Sitting, the eyes are closed and focused at the brow point. Raise your bent right knee up and place your right foot flat on the ground, toes pointing straight ahead. The sole of your left foot rests against the arch and ankle of your right foot. The ball of the left foot rests in front of the right ankle bone. Your left hand is in a fist by your left hip pressed into the floor for balance. Your right elbow is bent and resting on your right knee, while your right hand is cupped. It makes contact with the skull below the ear but stays open above the ear, as if you formed a cup of the hand to amplify a faint sound you want to hear.

Mantra – Inhale deeply. Chant in a long smooth sound as if someone is listening. Use a comfortable high pitch. *MAAAAAAAAAAAAAAAAAAAA* until you run out of breath. As you chant, listen to the sound. Hold your concentration on the sound and feel it vibrate through your whole body. I f you chant in a group, hear the overtones that develop and let those tones vibrate all around you and in every cell of your body. Continue for 11-31 minutes. Then change the legs and ear to the other side. Continue for an equal amount of time. Start slowly. Learn to hold the concentration into the sound. Build the meditation on each side to total 62 minutes.

midsummer solstice

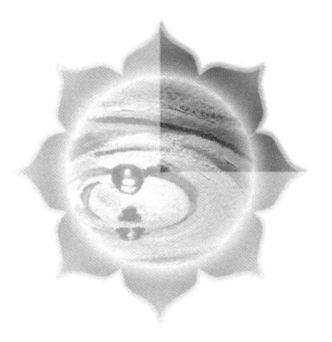

Reminders
- *Tune in to begin (page 53).*
- *Use the Neck Lock (page 16) in all postures unless otherwise stated.*
- *Unless otherwise stated, the mantra **Sat Nam** can be used during all exercises with each breath by silently vibrating Sat on the inhale and Nam on the exhale. End each exercise by inhaling deeply and applying the Root Lock (page 15) with the breath held in for 5- 15 seconds. Exhale.*
- *Close your session by singing **Longtime Sunshine** and chanting one long **Sat Nam.***

KRIYA

Abdominal Strengthening

This kriya gives you a good physical workout. It is excellent for your digestive system, improves circulation and strengthens your nervous system. It strengthens your navel point, abdominal muscles and lower back. It purifies your behavior so you become constant and direct.

Fire, summer, red, spirit, creativity, vision, South, Earth, flowers, lush with heat.

Fire that purifies and destroys, directing sight and creative vision to make things manifest in the world.

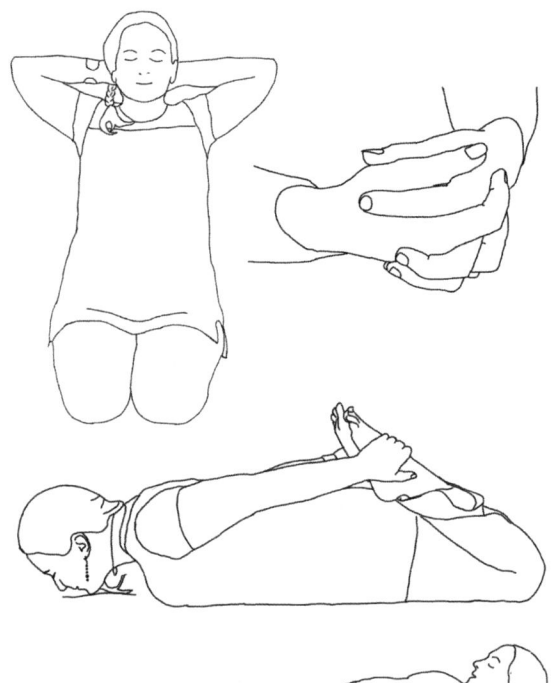

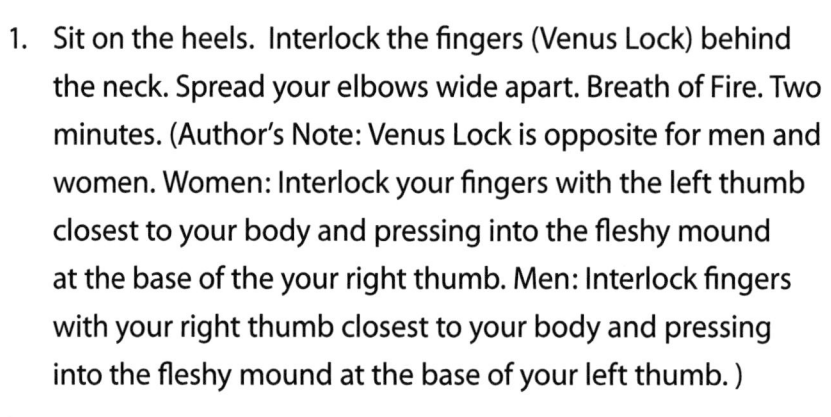

1. Sit on the heels. Interlock the fingers (Venus Lock) behind the neck. Spread your elbows wide apart. Breath of Fire. Two minutes. (Author's Note: Venus Lock is opposite for men and women. Women: Interlock your fingers with the left thumb closest to your body and pressing into the fleshy mound at the base of the your right thumb. Men: Interlock fingers with your right thumb closest to your body and pressing into the fleshy mound at the base of your left thumb.)

2. Lie on the stomach. Reach back and grab the ankles. Pull the ankles toward the buttocks keeping the chest on the ground. Hold for two minutes with normal breathing.

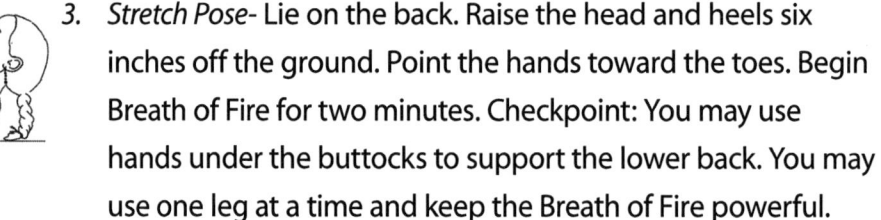

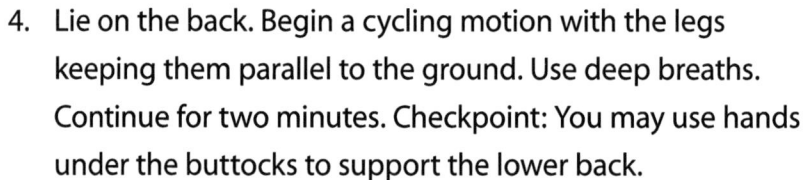

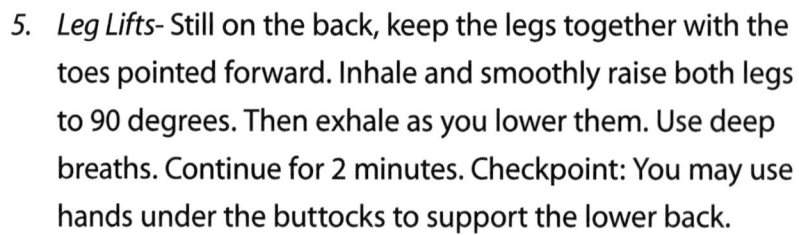

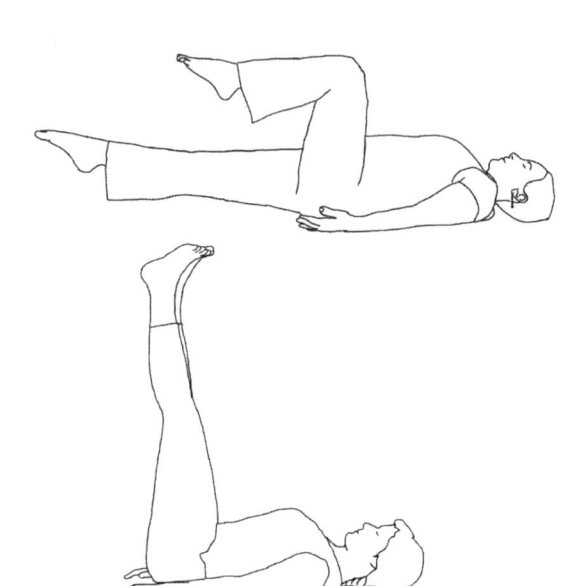

3. *Stretch Pose-* Lie on the back. Raise the head and heels six inches off the ground. Point the hands toward the toes. Begin Breath of Fire for two minutes. Checkpoint: You may use hands under the buttocks to support the lower back. You may use one leg at a time and keep the Breath of Fire powerful.

4. Lie on the back. Begin a cycling motion with the legs keeping them parallel to the ground. Use deep breaths. Continue for two minutes. Checkpoint: You may use hands under the buttocks to support the lower back.

5. *Leg Lifts-* Still on the back, keep the legs together with the toes pointed forward. Inhale and smoothly raise both legs to 90 degrees. Then exhale as you lower them. Use deep breaths. Continue for 2 minutes. Checkpoint: You may use hands under the buttocks to support the lower back.

6. Lie on the stomach. Place the palms on the ground under the shoulders. Slowly arch up into Cobra Pose. Lift the feet up toward the head. Hold for two minutes.

Author's note: Place the hands under the shoulders with fingers spread wide and the heels touching. Apply Mulbandh and gently let your breath lead the movement. Arch your upper back, pulling the shoulders down and back, stretching up and away from the lower back. Open the heart, lift the chest and head, and if you are flexible, let the head gently fall back and straighten the arms, keeping the arms close to the body. Do not over-stretch!

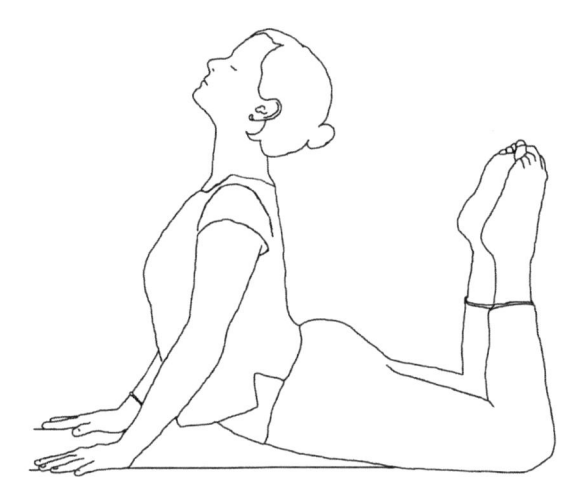

Author's modification: Rest on the forearms and keep the elbows bent.

7. Lie on the back. Bring both knees up to the chest and hold them there with the hands. Roll forward and back on the spine. Continue for two minutes.

8. Lie on the stomach. Extend the arms forward with the palms flat together. Arch the back so the arms, chest and legs lift off the ground. Hold this Extended Locust with Breath of Fire for two minutes.

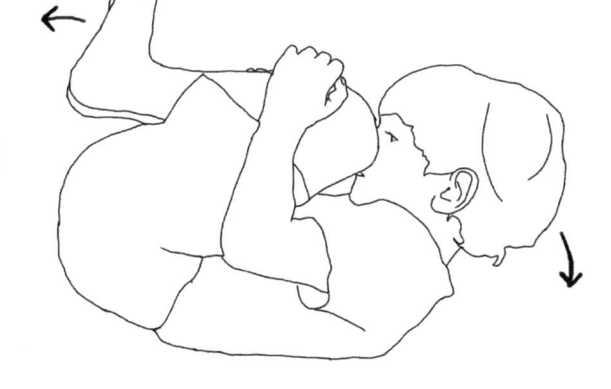

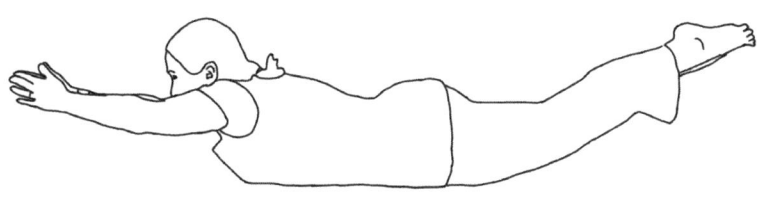

Author's note: Feel your lower back elongating as you reach forward with your arms and stretch backwards with your legs, as if being pulled in both directions.

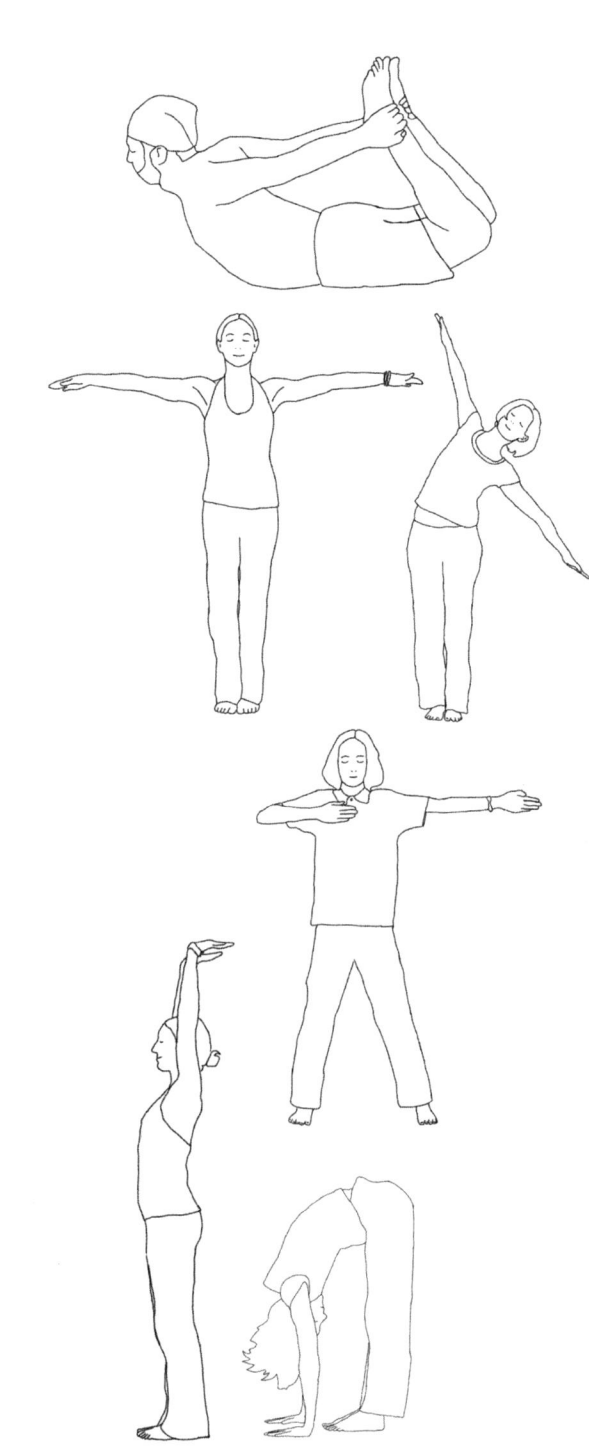

9. Still on the stomach, reach back and grasp the ankles. Arch up into Bow Pose. Do Breath of Fire for two minutes then relax.

Author's note: Press the ankles into the palms. Author's Modification: If you can't reach your ankles, reach towards them. Arch up and visualize the posture.

10. Stand up straight. Keep legs together. Extend the arms to the sides, parallel to the ground with palms facing down. Without twisting the torso, bend to the left with a deep inhale, then bend to the right with the exhale. Continue this pendulum-like motion for two minutes.

Author's note: Place the feet together with toes and heels touching, and weight evenly distributed with thighs moving inward to open the sacrum. Apply Mulbandh and Neck Lock. Rhythmically as you bend, stretch along the sides of the rib cage, opening the ribs.

11. Still standing, spread the legs 1 ½ to 2 feet apart. Then swing one arm out to the side, parallel to the ground as the other arm bends in with the palm on the chest. Then switch arms. Inhale as the left arm swings out, exhale as the right arm swings out. Continue for 2 minutes

12. Still standing, raise both arms straight up with palms facing up. Exhale as you bend forward and try to put the palms on the ground. Inhale as you raise up. Continue for two minutes.

Author's note: Lift the chest and gently arch back, pressing shoulder blades down. On the exhale, bend forward from the navel point, bringing your palms to the floor. As you continue bending and rising, allow the breath to initiate the movement. Author's Modification: If you can't touch the floor, reach towards it. If there is discomfort in the lower back, bend your knees.

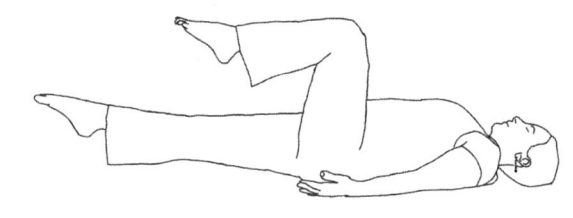

13. Lie on the back. Repeat the 4th exercise, Parallel Bicycle, for 2 minutes.

14. On the back, inhale while raising the left leg to 90 degrees. Exhale as you lower it. Repeat with the right leg. For 2 minutes, continue this alternate leg lifting with deep breaths.

Author's note: use the navel as a brake to lower the leg down.

15. Sit on the heels with the arms stretched up and the palms together. Begin Sat Kriya. Pull in the navel point and say SAT, relax the navel point and say NAM. Continue rhythmically for two minutes. Then inhale deeply, hold and apply Mulbandh. Relax.

Author's note: Refer to Sat Kriya (page 83).

16. Sit straight with both legs extended. Lift the legs up 60 degrees from the ground. Extend the arms parallel to the ground with palms down. Begin Breath of Fire. Continue for 2 minutes. Then totally relax.

Author's note: Do not collapse the chest; keep the heart open and lifted, with shoulder blades moving down the back. Author's Modifications: Grasp hold of the legs. Bend the knees.

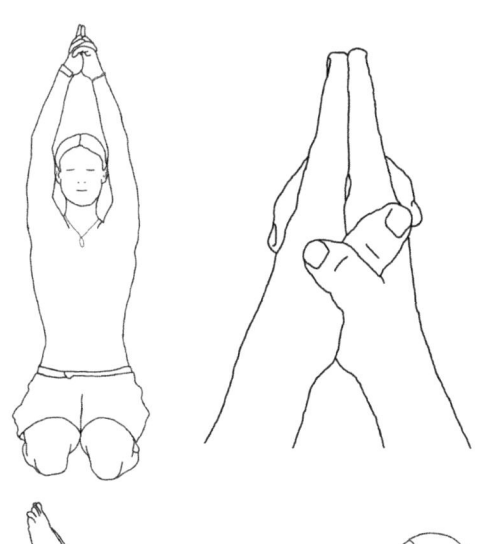

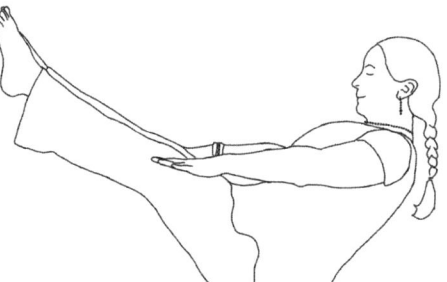

KRIYA

Strengthening the Aura

This kriya develops your aura and helps keep disease away. It extends the power of protection from outside influences and disease and extends your projection or clarity of intention in your personality. When practiced regularly and with full times, a tremendous healing sweat is produced, and it is said to cure almost any digestive problem.

1. *Yogic Push-Ups*

    Stand up. Bend forward, placing the hands on the floor in Triangle Pose (Downward Dog) so that your body forms a triangle. Inhale. Raise your right leg up with knee straight. Exhale and bend the arms. Bring the head near the floor. Inhale and rise up to the original position. Exhale down. Continue the push-ups, bending only the elbows. 1 ½ - 7 ½ minutes. Stand up, take a few deep breaths and switch legs. Repeat for same amount of time.

2. *Arm Raises*

    Sit in Easy Pose. Extend left arm forward as if shaking hands. Bring your right hand underneath your left and grasp the back of your left hand with your right so both palms face right and your fingers lock. Inhale and raise your arms up 60° above horizontal. Exhale and bring the arms back down to chest level. Continue this chopping rhythm with powerful breaths for 2-15 minutes. To end, inhale with arms up. Exhale. Relax.

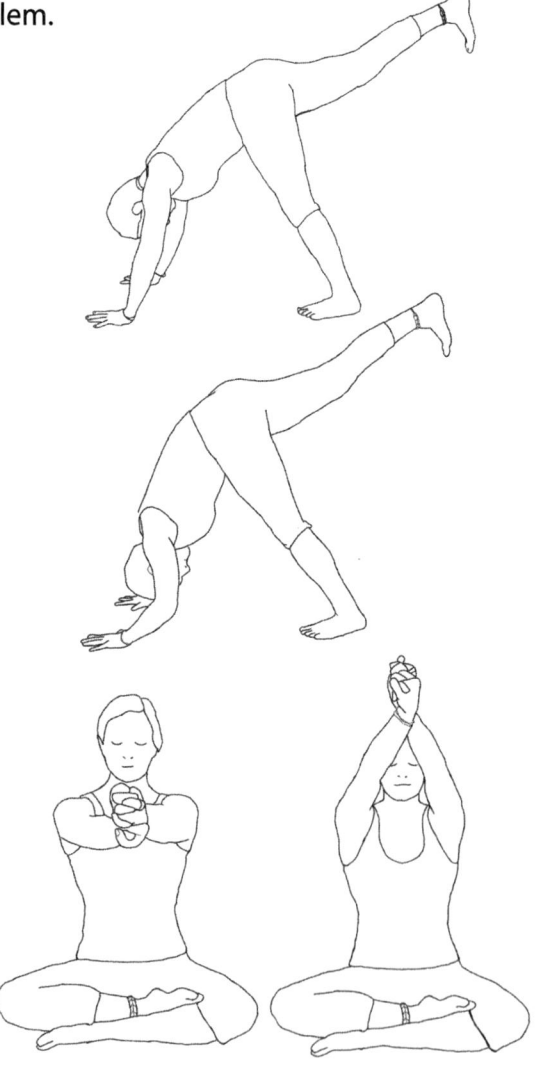

3. Sit in Easy Pose. Extend both arms forward, parallel to the floor, with palms 6 inches apart and facing each other. Inhale, open the arms back, stretching towards each other. Exhale and bring arms back to the original position. Powerful rhythmic breaths. Visualize your arms moving the aura in ripples, then extend your aura further out for 2-15 minutes.

Meditation

Karnee (Creativity) Kriya | Originally taught on May 17, 1979.

Yogi Bhajan said about this meditation, "Discipline of the consciousness is the acknowledgement of the spirit. All human difficulties can be eliminated once you have a harmony between conscious mind and subconscious mind toward the supreme conscious mind…Harmony between conscious and subconscious is a gateway to Infinity and that is the spirit we are talking about."

Sit in Easy Pose with a straight spine. Bend the Sun (ring) and Mercury (pinky) fingers and lock them down with your thumbs. Extend your Saturn (middle) and Jupiter (index) fingers. Touch the tips of your Jupiter fingers together and the tips of the Saturn fingers together, keeping your fingers as straight as possible. Hold this mudra at chin level with your arms parallel to the floor.

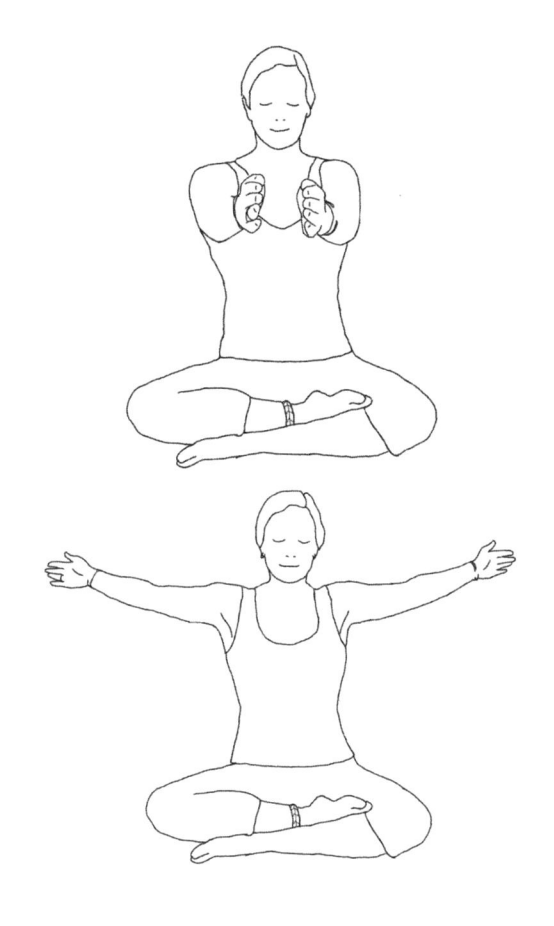

1. Try to keep your eyes open.

2. Inhale, quickly and deeply, for two or three seconds. Hold your breath as long as you comfortably can, at least five seconds. Mentally recite any mantra of your choice while you hold your breath.

3. Exhale slowly and completely, 10 to 15 seconds. Continue this breathing pattern for 11 minutes.

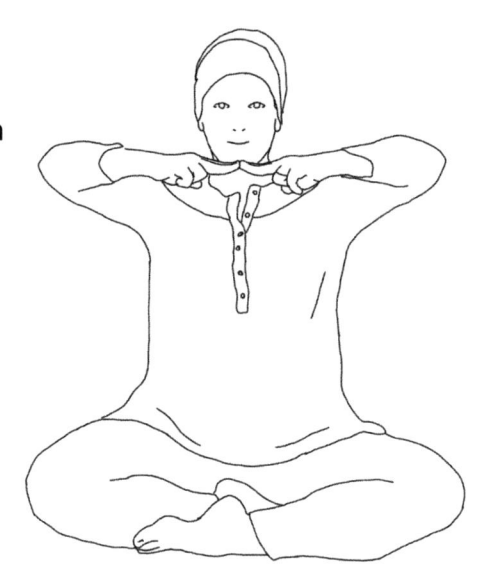

Chanting as Singing and Devotion

Bhaja Man Mere

This chant celebrates devotional singing to bring your lower mind or ego to the wisdom and ecstasy of love, beauty and the Divine. Your mind is delivered to its true identity of Infinite Self as human experience. May be chanted anytime.

Bhaja Man Mere Hari Ka Nam Hari Ka Nam Sat Nam

1. Sit with a straight spine, hands in Gyan Mudra, eyes closed, chant for three or more minutes.

2. To end, sit in stillness and notice the resonance vibrating in every cell of your body. Notice who is noticing.

The instructions for this meditation are from the CD *Angel's Waltz* by Sada Sat Kaur Khalsa and could not be verified by *KRI Review*.

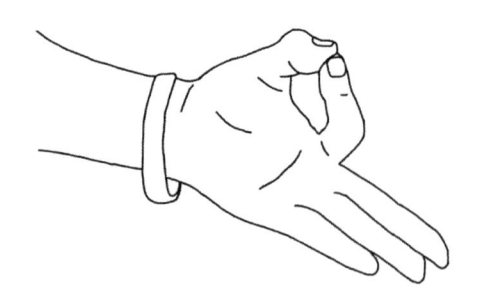

autumn equinox

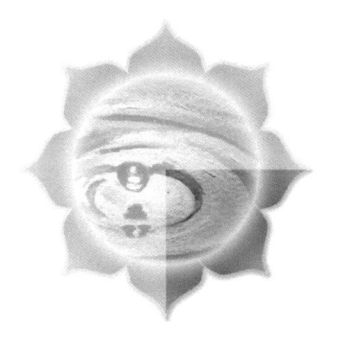

Reminders
- Tune in to begin (page 53).
- Use the Neck Lock (page 16) in all postures unless otherwise stated.
- Unless otherwise stated, the mantra **Sat Nam** can be used during all exercises with each breath by silently vibrating Sat on the inhale and Nam on the exhale. End each exercise by inhaling deeply and applying the Root Lock (page 15) with the breath held in for 5- 15 seconds. Exhale.
- Close your session by singing **Longtime Sunshine** and chanting one long **Sat Nam**.

KRIYA

Pituitary Gland Series

This set of exercises gives a complete workout for your pituitary gland, which then stimulates the other master glands to strengthen your immune system.

Water, autumn, blue, emotions, intuition, psychic abilities, West.

A time of fullness and maturity, marks time of harvest and completion of vegetation cycle. Light and warmth declines.

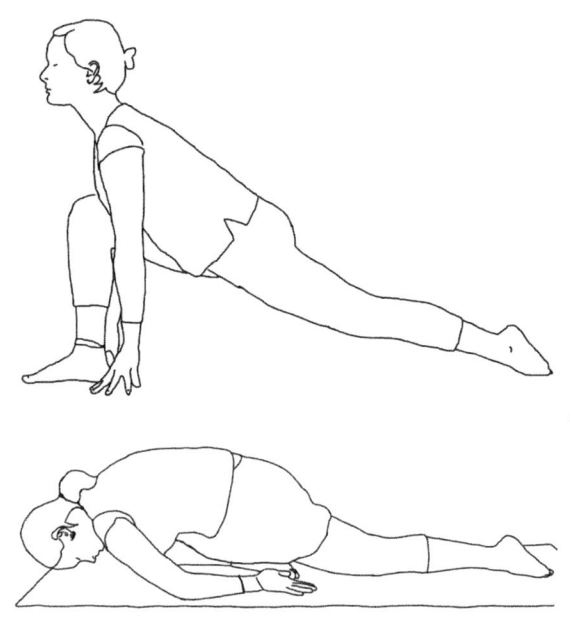

1. **Lunge Stretch**
   Bend the right knee with the right foot flat on the floor. Extend the left leg straight back and place the hands on the floor for balance. Arch the head back and hold the position, breathing slowly and deeply for one minute. Then do Breath of Fire for two minutes.

2. **Lunge Stretch Rest**
   From position #1, bring the right knee down to the floor and bend the torso to rest over the thigh. Place forehead on the floor, stretch the left leg all the way back and rest the arms by the sides, palms up. Breathe slowly and deeply three minutes.

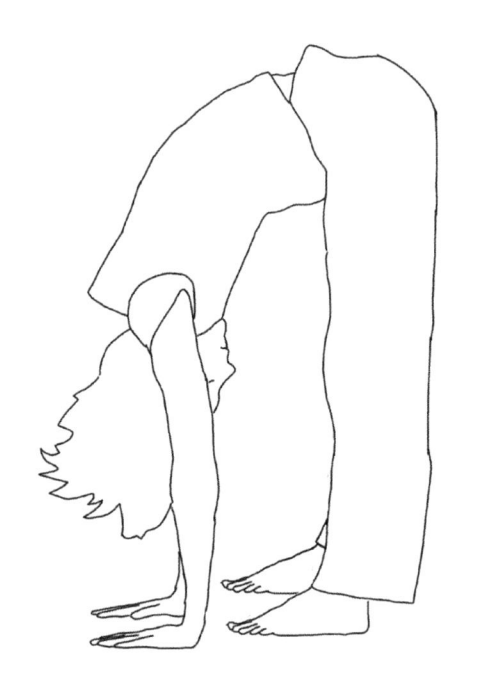

3. Repeat exercises 1 and 2 with the opposite legs.

4. **Front Bend**
   Stand up with the feet about two feet apart apart. Bend over and touch the fingertips or the palms on the floor. Do long deep breathing for three minutes.

Author's note: Begin by inhaling deeply as you expand your ribs, lifting the spine up. On the exhale, draw the navel point in and up, bend forward hinged from the hips, lifting and lengthening forward from the navel point, keeping your spine as straight as possible. The head gently follows last. Reverse to come up, pushing feet into the floor, head follows last.

5. **Ego Eradicator**

   Stand up again and stretch the arms overhead at a 30 degree angle, thumbs pointing up, fingers on the palms. Keep your elbows straight as you breathe long and deeply for three minutes.

Checkpoints: When seated in Easy Pose for Ego Eradicator, the arms are stretched overhead at a 60 degree angle. When standing for Ego Eradicator, the angle is 30 degrees, as pictured, for balance.

6. **Triangle Pose** (AKA Downward Dog)

   Come onto the hands and knees and push up into Triangle Pose. The heels are flat on the floor and the head and neck relax. Hold for up to three minutes.

Author's note: Lift the hips up so the body forms a triangle. Fingers are spread wide with middle fingers pointing straight ahead. Allow the underarms to face each other. Try to bring the heels to the floor. Arms and legs are straight. Look toward the feet or knees. Feel the thighs move towards the wall behind you. With each inhale, push into the palms. With each exhale, lift the tailbone.)

7. **Cobra Pose**

   Relax on the stomach for one minute. Then bring the heels together, palms flat on the floor under the shoulders. Push up into Cobra Pose. Stretch the head and neck back and begin Long Deep Breathing for one minute. Then turn the head from side to side, inhaling to the left, exhaling to the right. Continue for two minutes. Inhale, exhale and pull Mulbandh three times.

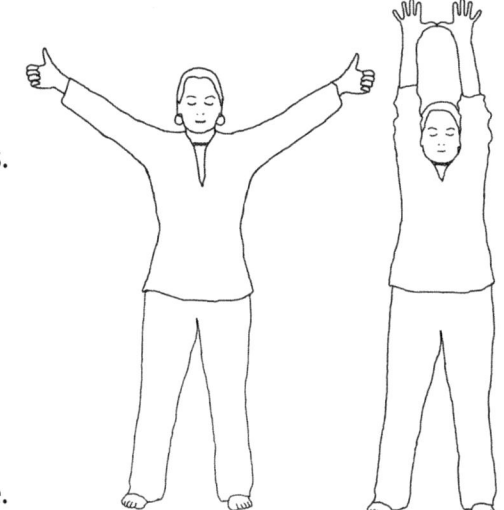

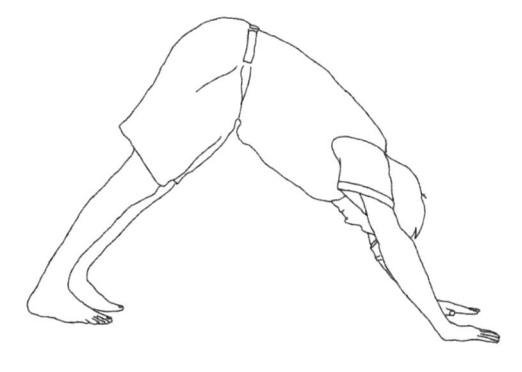

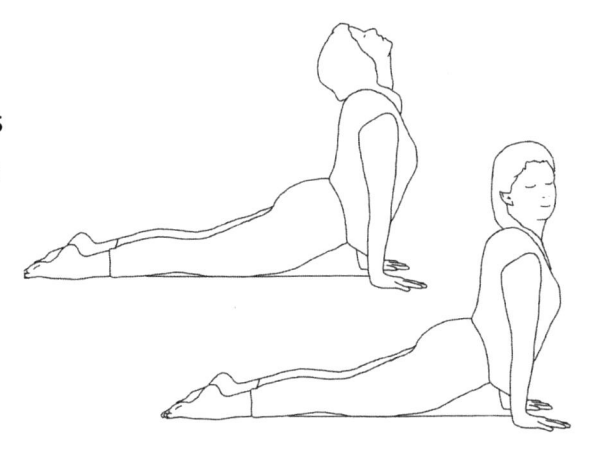

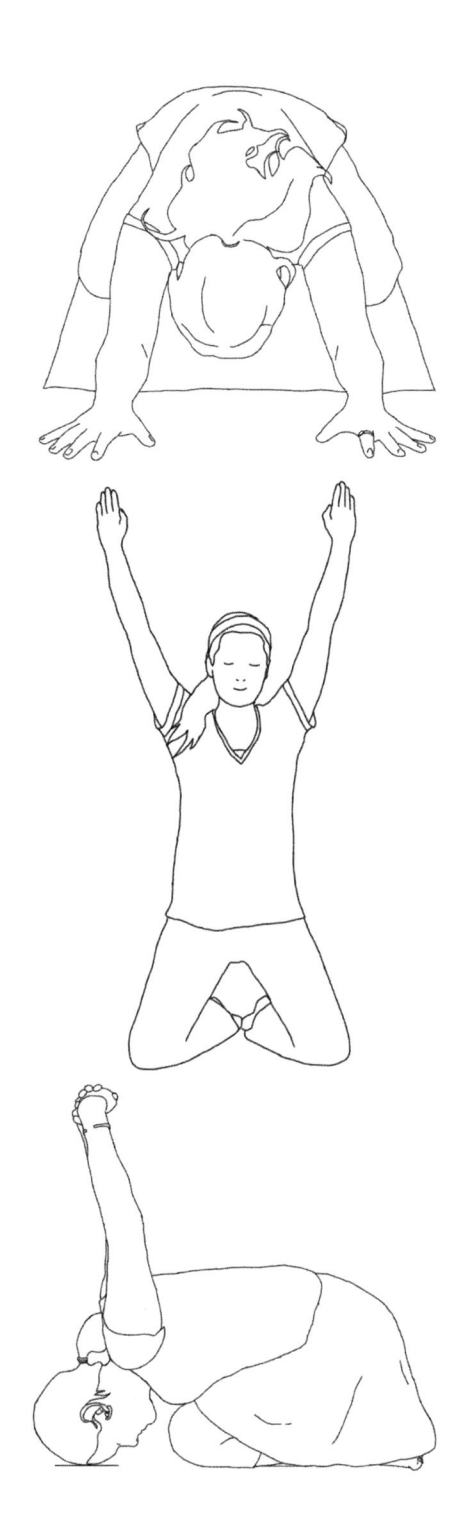

8. **Rock Pose**

    Sit on the heels in Rock Pose and spread the knees far apart. Bring the forehead to the floor with the palms flat on the floor in front of the knees. Inhale and rise up on the knees, stretching the arms up and out like a flower greeting the sun. Exhale and come down bringing the forehead to the floor. Continue for three minutes.

Author's modification: You can place a pillow or rolled up blankets in front of you to shorten the distance your forehead travels to the floor.

9. **Yoga Mudra**

    Sit on the heels again with the knees together and the fingers interlaced at the base of the spine. Bring the forehead to the ground and lift the arms up straight as far as possible and hold the position for three minutes with Long Deep Breathing.

Author's modification: You can place a pillow or rolled up blankets in front of you to shorten the distance your forehead travels to the floor.

Meditation

Creative Meditation of the Sublime Self | Originally Taught February 12, 1976.

Exercise and warm-up for the meditation

This exercise clears out the lymph glands in the upper chest, makes the heart healthy and is good for the breast area. It works on the left and right hemispheres of the brain, creating a balance between them. It will make you quick to know what to do.

1. Sit calmly in a comfortable position. Relax your arms at your sides with your palms facing forward. Alternately bend each elbow, bringing your palms toward the center of your chest, but do not touch your chest. Do not bend your wrists or hands. Move as rapidly as you can. You should have sweat on your forehead after a couple of minutes. Maintain a balance in the rhythmic motion of your hands. If your hands hit each other, it means that this balance is upset.

As a warm-up for the following meditation, practice this exercise for 3-11 minutes. (If you practice this exercise on its own, do it for 10 or 15 minutes every morning.)

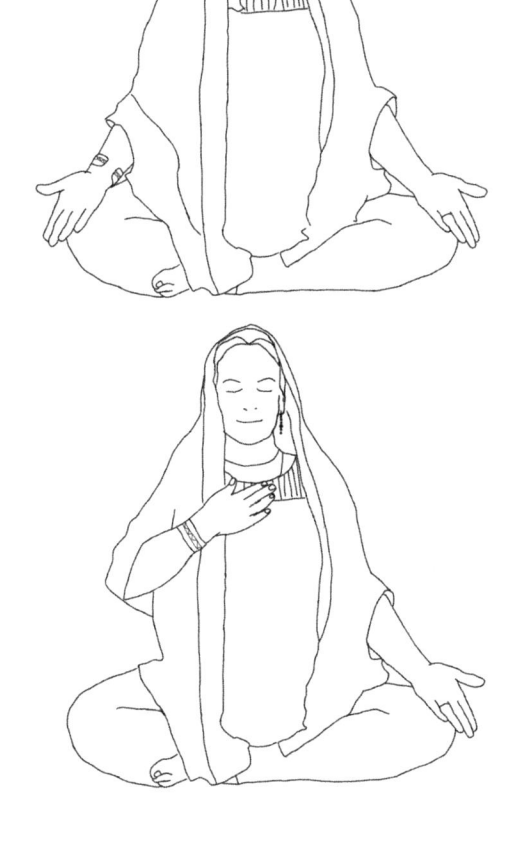

Meditation

2. Immediately after practicing the warm-up, with your elbows still at your sides, bring your forearms up to 60 degrees. Place the sides of the hands together, palms up, at the height of the diaphragm. The fingers are relaxed and spread slightly. The thumbs are relaxed and slightly up and out.

    Look right into the center of the hands, where the Mercury (pinky) fingers are. Inhale deeply and chant HARIANG 8 times on one breath. Each chanting cycle takes about 10 seconds.

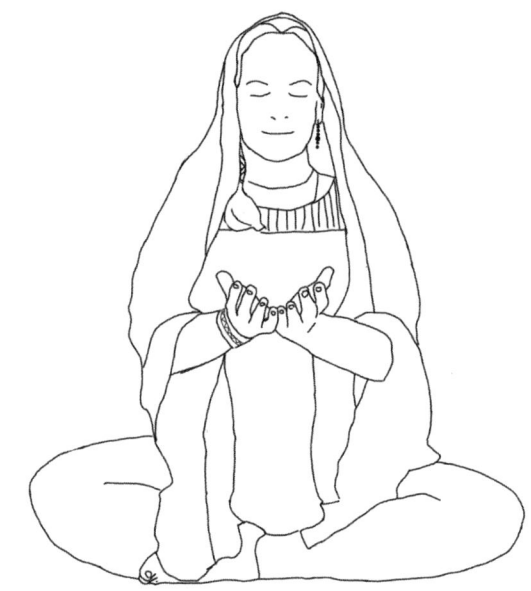

    HARIANG means *Shiva, Destroyer of Evil*. It is a powerful mantra, which brings wealth and intuitive opportunity. When chanting HARIANG, the tip of the tongue touches the roof of the mouth behind the front teeth to make the "R" sound.

    It may take a couple of months to bring this meditation under your control, but if you do this meditation for 90 days, it will activate your brain so that you will know exactly what is what. It will make you super sensitive. It will make it intuitively possible for you to live creatively to your own potential and to tap into the opportunities around you.

Checkpoints: There are 84 points in the upper part of the mouth and the tongue works like acupressure. When you speak, the tongue touches those areas and stimulates the nervous system and brain. The words we call mantra are designed to stimulate a particular combination of meridians in the mouth. These words also have a projective power. The theory is that the huge computer mind is infinite and our mind is limited. If you know the combination of the frequency of the signal, which can tap the resources of the Infinite Mind, then the flow of Infinity will start appearing to your finite mind. Mantra is nothing but a telecommunication of the finite unto the Infinite. The individual creates a frequency of vibration within his electro-magnetic field to tap the electro-magnetic field of the Universe.

Meditation

The Ancient Way Of Prayer | Originally Taught October 8, 1979.

Yogi Bhajan said about this meditation, "It is a simple prayer, the oldest manner of prayer ever known to mankind."

Sit in Easy Pose with a straight spine. Rest the elbows against the ribs with the forearms angled out to the sides and the palms facing upward. The forearms angle up so that the hands are at the level of the heart center. The fingers of each hand are joined, the thumbs are a little spread and the hands are relaxed and receptive. It is a very relaxed and comfortable hand and arm position.

Concentrate between the eyebrows and the root of the nose. Inhale deeply, exhale completely, hold the breath out, and tune in to the beat of the heart, mentally vibrating THOU with each beat. Hold the breath for 15-30 seconds. "Silently listen to the beat of the heart, which silently chants THOU, THOU, THOU. Meditate on the beautiful, rhythmic beat of your own heart." Yogi Bhajan.

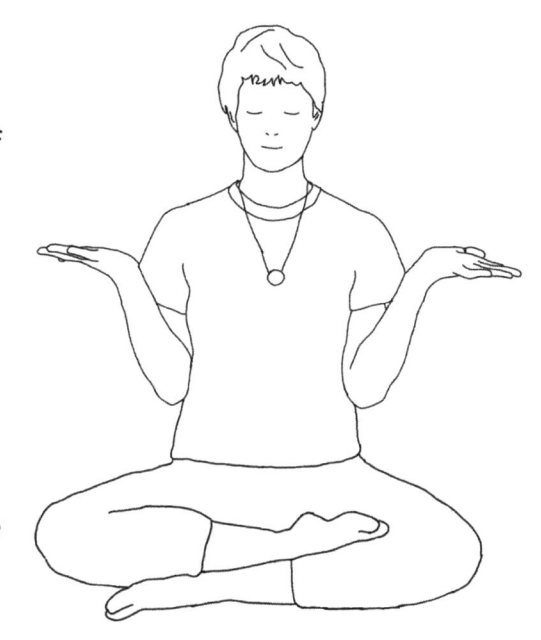

Continue this breath pattern. Begin with 11 minutes and develop your practice to half an hour.

You may find that you are not in a position to tune in to the heartbeat and hear "Thou" with each beat, so there is an alternative way to time the practice of this meditation: Inhale deeply, exhale completely and mentally chant *SAA-TAA-NAA-MAA* four times with the breath held out. The mantra will give you a similar timing and rhythm to your heartbeat, if each syllable is mentally vibrated once per second. (Four repetitions of SAA-TAA-NAA-MAA will take about sixteen seconds.) Continue this breath pattern. Begin with eleven minutes and develop your practice to half an hour.

It is important that the breath is held out of the lungs for the same amount of time throughout the meditation; therefore, you must mentally vibrate the mantra at a consistent rate.

Yogi Bhajan said, "It is a simple prayer, the oldest manner of prayer ever known to mankind. It is said in the Scriptures that an individual can control his own death and the death of others through the correct practice of this kriya. There are about three pages telling what this kriya does for you, but I can't relate all that. But, at the end of the third page, underlined, the punch line is that such a person can have control over his own death, which they say is not controllable. And can control the death of others. And for people like us, who live in America, who cannot control their communications and live always in doubt and misery, I think this will be an added attraction."

Chanting Meditation

Sat Narayan | Sat Narayan Wahe Guru Hari Narayan Sat Nam

This chant creates a strong heart without breaking the heart. It vibrates the thymus gland. It means *Indescribable is the ecstasy of the truth, the wisdom, that I am preserved and sustained by unity with absolute reality*. Narayan is a name of God as sustainer and preserver. It is the name of Vishnu.

1. Sit comfortably with a straight spine. Eyes closed.

2. Mudra: Right hand, Gyan Mudra. Left hand, 4 inches out from your body at the heart in heart shield. Fingers point to the right. 3-11 minutes. This is a very powerful and effective chanting meditation. Do not exceed 11 minutes in a 24-hour period.

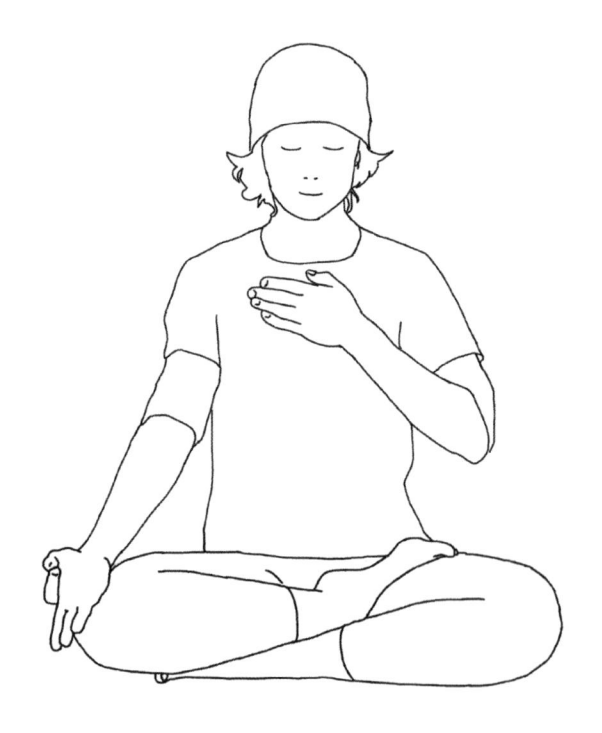

midwinter solstice

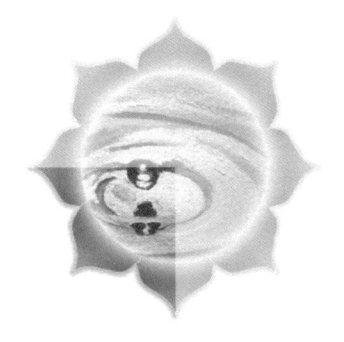

Reminders
- *Tune in to begin (page 53).*
- *Use the Neck Lock (page 16) in all postures unless otherwise stated.*
- *Unless otherwise stated, the mantra* **Sat Nam** *can be used during all exercises with each breath by silently vibrating Sat on the inhale and Nam on the exhale. End each exercise by inhaling deeply and applying the Root Lock (page 15) with the breath held in for 5-15 seconds. Exhale.*
- *Close your session by singing* **Longtime Sunshine** *and chanting one long* **Sat Nam.**

KRIYA

Self-Adjustment of the Spine

Make sure to warm-up before practicing this kriya. This set of exercises works to create a well-adjusted spine, flexible with relaxed muscles.

Earth, winter, green, material things, physical plane, North.

Sun is reborn when the earth sleeps. Days and light lengthen. Promise of spring and regeneration. Money and the manifest world that supports us and nourishes us. Experiencing power of touch.

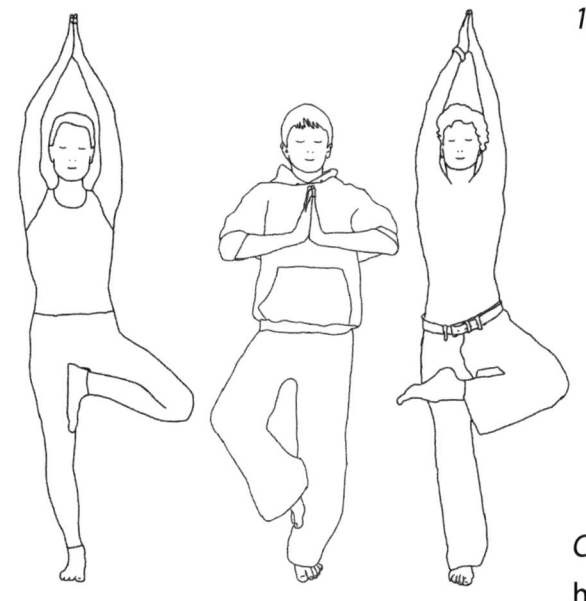

1. **Tree Pose**

    From a standing position, raise your left leg and place your foot alongside your upper thigh with your toes pointing downward. Bring your palms together at the heart in Prayer Mudra. Eyes are open and focused on one spot in front of you. This will help you balance. Keep your hands in Prayer Pose and raise them up overhead, maintaining a constant upward pull. Gently press your bent knee backward to straighten the spine further. Breathe long and deeply. One to two minutes. Switch legs.

    Checkpoints: If you are more flexible, place your raised left heel against your pubic bone with the sole of your foot facing slightly upward with your toes pointing toward your right hip. This is ideal because this will cause pressure at the base of your spine and all your vertebrae will adjust accordingly. Continue and then switch legs.

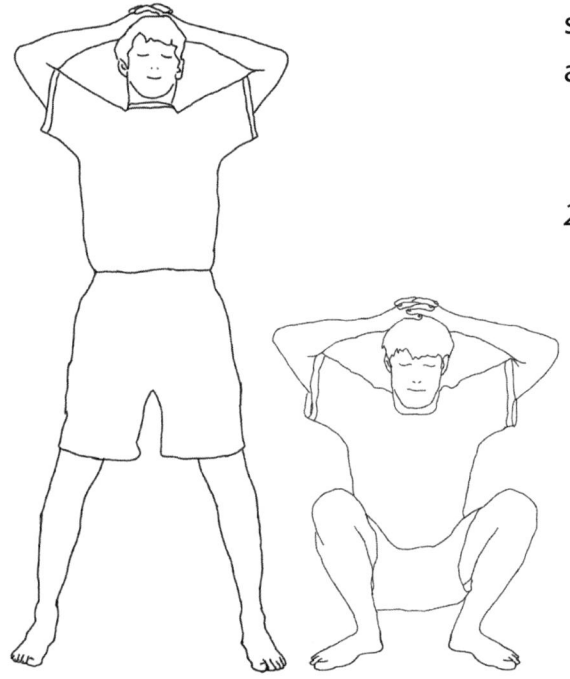

2. **Crow Squats**

    Stand straight. Inhale and apply Neck Lock (Chin in, chest out). Interlock your fingers and place them on the top of your head. Exhale, squat down with your knees and feet wide apart and your heels flat on the floor, if possible. Keep your knees over your feet. Continue inhaling up to beginning position and exhaling down into Crow Squat. Use powerful breaths that initiate the movement. One to two minutes. (Author's note: When teaching, I instruct students to keep it real! Squat only as far as you are able.)

3. *Chair Bounce*

   Come into Chair Pose with feet shoulder-width apart and knees bent with back and thighs parallel to floor. Hands come through your legs and around the back of your heels to grasp the tops of your feet. If that is not possible, grasp your heels. Look down. Bounce the lower back and buttocks up (inhale) and down (exhale) 11 times. Slowly stand up, breathe normally for 5 seconds. Then come back into chair and resume bouncing and standing pattern for 2-3 minutes. Relax for 30 seconds in Easy Pose.

4. *Side Stretches*

   Stand up straight and spread your legs apart as far as possible, to maintain balance. Extend your arms straight out to the sides with palms facing down. Bend to the right and stretch your right arm toward the right foot. Your left arm stretches upward. Gaze at the left hand. Hold for 10 seconds. Without stopping, slowly and smoothly switch sides. Keep your arms in a straight unbroken line throughout the exercise. Continue 1-3 minutes.

5. Relax in Corpse Pose.

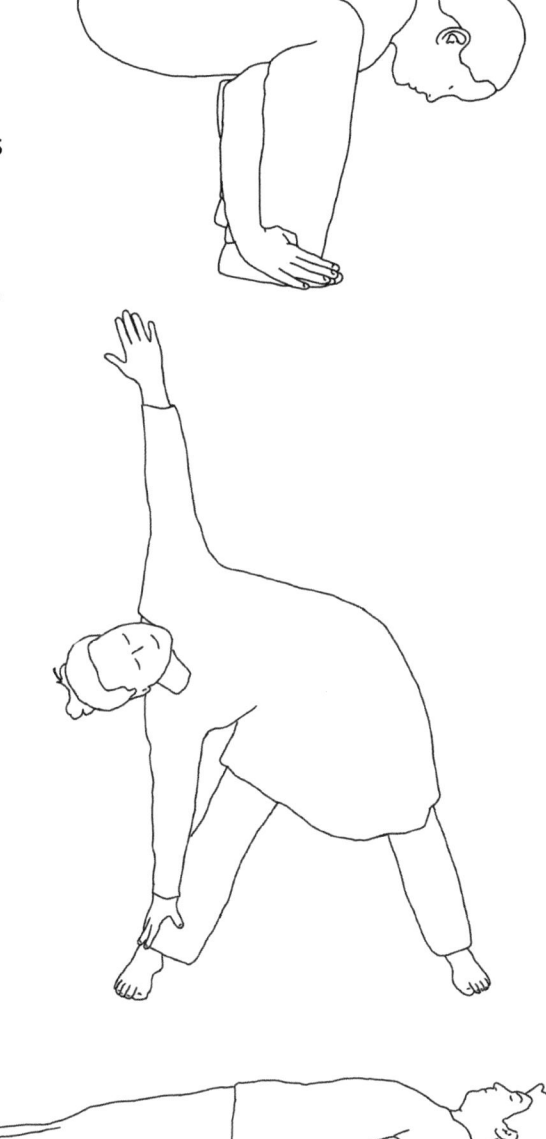

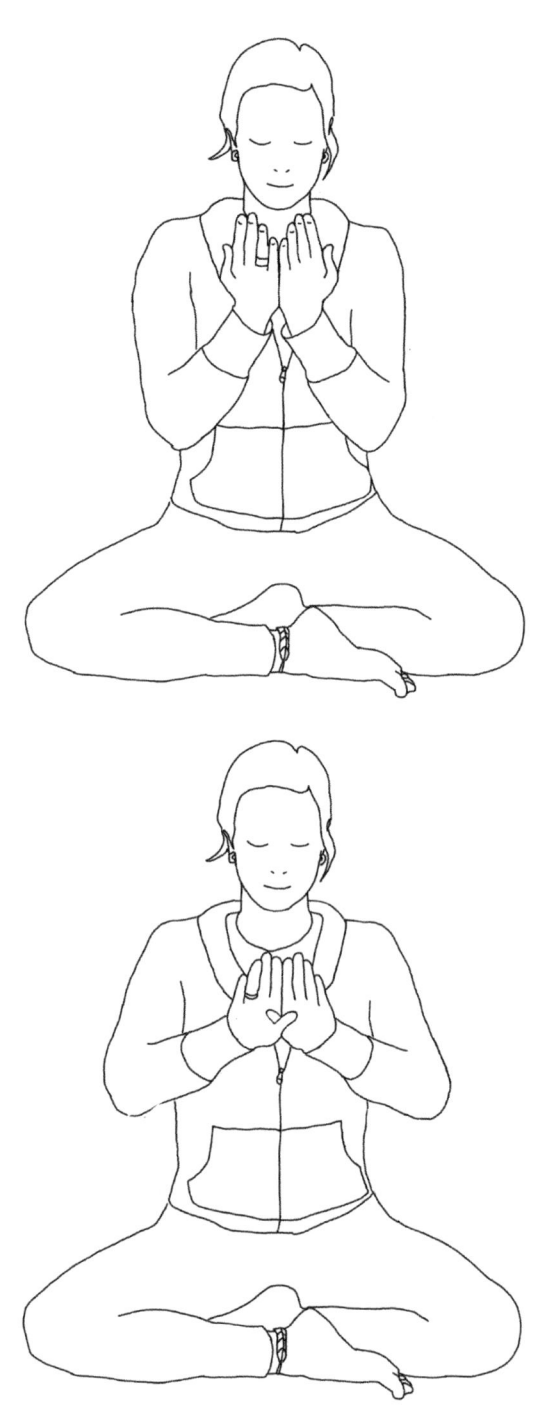

KRIYA

Subagh Kriya | Originally Taught June 21, 1996.

This is a 5 part kriya. Each part must be practiced for an equal amount of time, either 3 minutes or 11 minutes. Do not exceed 11 minutes. Only the first exercise of this kriya may be practiced on its own, separately from the other exercises.

1. Sit in Easy Pose with a straight spine. Allow your upper arms to be relaxed, with the elbows bent and the palms in front of the chest. Strike the outer sides of the hands together, forcefully hitting the area from the base of the little finger (Mercury Finger) to the base of the palm. This area is called the Moon area. Next turn the palms to face down and strike the sides of the index fingers (Jupiter fingers) together. Alternately strike the Moon area and the Jupiter area as you chant HAR with the tip of your tongue, pulling the navel with each HAR. Your eyes are focused at the tip of your nose. This meditation was taught to the rhythm of Tantric Har by Simran Kaur.

Yogi Bhajan said, " I'm going to give you a very handy tool, one that you can use anywhere, and you'll become rich. To become rich and prosperous, with wealth and values, is to have the strength to come through. It means that transmissions from your brain and the power of your intuition can immediately tell you what to do."

2. Stretch your arms out to the sides and up at a sixty-degree angle. Spread your fingers wide, making them stiff. The palms face forward. Cross your arms in front of your face. Alternate the position of the arms as they cross: first the left arm crosses in front of the right and then the right arm crosses in front of the left. Continue crossing the arms, keeping the elbows straight and the fingers open and stiff. This movement is also done to the rhythm of Tantric Har by Simran Kaur, but this time you do not chant.

3. Keep your arms out and up at sixty degrees as in the previous exercise. With your hands make a fist around your thumb, squeezing your thumb tightly as if you are trying to squeeze all the blood out of it. Move your arms in small backward circles as you continue squeezing your thumb. Your arms are stretched and the elbows stay straight. Chant the mantra GOD powerfully from your navel. One backward circle of the arms equals one repetition of GOD. The speed and rhythm of the chanting is the same as in the previous exercises. Move powerfully so that your entire spine shakes, you may even be lifted slightly up off the ground by the movement.

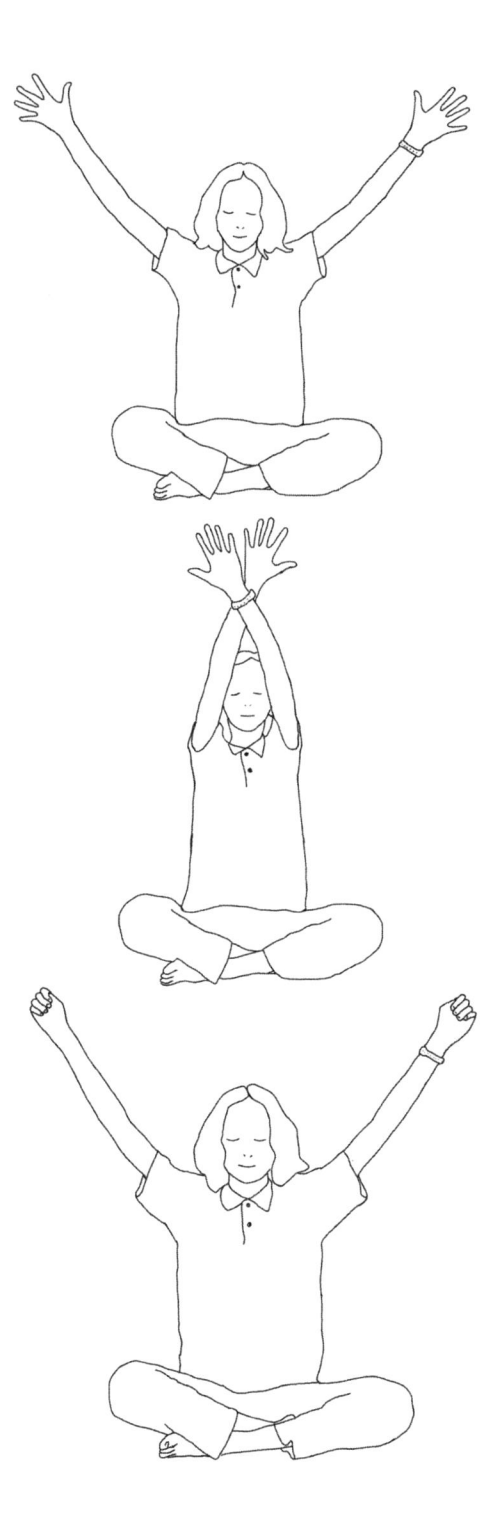

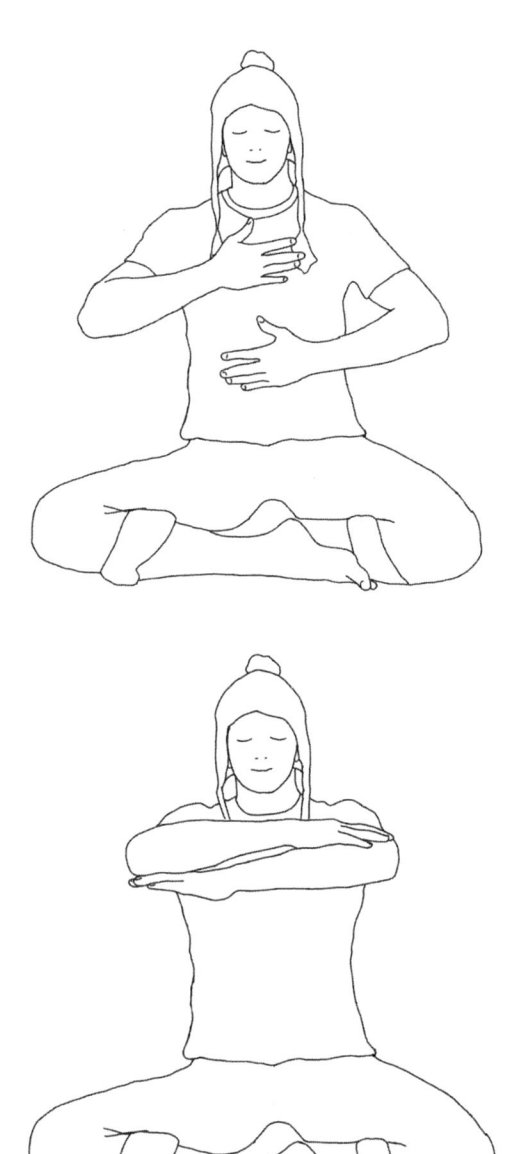

4. Bend your arms so that your elbows point to the sides. The forearms are parallel to the floor and the palms face the body around the level of the diaphragm. The right hand moves up a few inches as the left hand moves down. The left hand moves up as the right hand moves down. The hands move alternately up and down between the heart and navel. As the hands move, chant HAR HARAY HAREE, WHAHAY GURU in a deep monotone with one repetition of the mantra approximately every 4 seconds. Chant from your navel. If you are practicing the exercises for 11 minutes each, then you will chant the mantra out loud for 6 minutes, whisper it strongly for 3 minutes, and then whistle it for 2 minutes. If you are practicing the exercises for 3 minutes each, then you will chant the mantra out loud for 1 minute, whisper it strongly for 1 minute, and then whisper it for one minute.

5. Bend your elbows and rest your right forearm on your left forearm, with your palms down. The arms are held in front of your body at shoulder height. Close your eyes, keep your arms steady. Keep your spine straight and your arms parallel to the floor. Breathe slowly and deeply so that one breath takes a full minute. Inhale for 20 seconds, hold for 20 seconds, and exhale for 20 seconds.

note: About Subagh Kriya Yogi Bhajan has said, "It's a complete set. This is all called Subagh Kriya. If God has written with His own hands that you shall live under misfortune, then by doing Subagh Kriya you can turn misfortune into prosperity, fortune, and good luck."

Meditation

Burn Inner Anger | Originally Taught February 19, 2000.

Yogi Bhajan said about this meditation: Breathe strongly and powerfully with emotion. Burn your inner anger and get rid of it. Take the help of the breath to get rid of the body's weaknesses and impurities.
In 11 minutes' time, if you get into correct posture, breathing, and angle of the hand, it will re-build within you a very powerful immune system. If you do it every day, after 40 days you will be a different person. After 40 days of practice with the right hand extended, you may switch hands and do 40 days with the left arm extended and the right hand on the chest. After 40 days in this position, you may do another 40 days of both arms extended. This is how it goes (for those who want an extended practice). But start somewhere and start small. There is no place for over-doing in Kundalini Yoga.

1. Sit in Easy Pose with a straight spine, chin in and chest out. Extend the Jupiter and Saturn (index and middle) fingers of your right hand and use your thumb to hold down the other fingers. Raise your right arm in front and up to 60 degrees. Keep your elbow straight. Place your left hand at the heart center (the center of your chest). Close your eyes. Make an *O* of your mouth and inhale and exhale powerfully through your mouth. (2-second inhalation and 2-second exhalation) Continue for 11 minutes.

2. To finish, inhale deeply, hold the breath for 10 seconds, stretch both arms up over your head, and stretch your spine as much as you can. Stretch the discs between your vertebrae. Exhale like cannon fire. Repeat this breath sequence 2 more times.

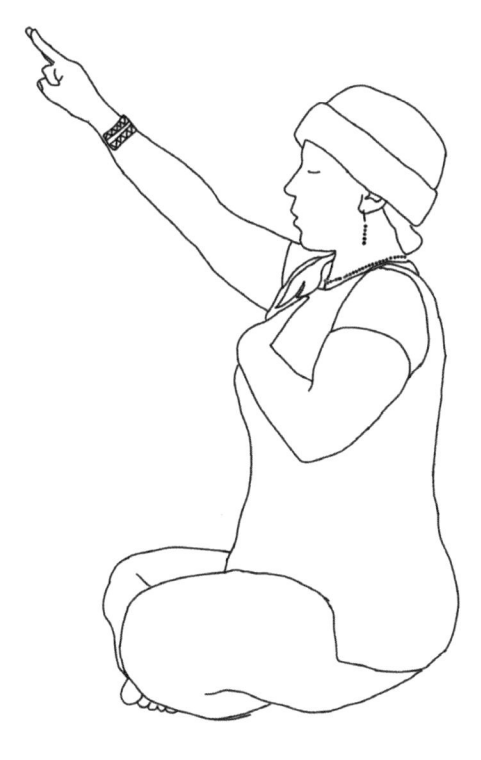

Chanting Meditation

Siri Gaitri Mantra | Originally taught in Summer 1973.

RA MA DA SA SA SAY SO HUNG

This ancient Sanskrit mantra is a rare and beautiful gem and is a powerful meditation for healing self and others. In this process of healing others, you are healed as well. It captures the radiant healing energy of the Cosmos. This mantra is called a *Sushmuna* Mantra. It has eight sounds that stimulate the Kundalini energy to flow into the central channel of the spine and in the chakras. This causes a metabolic change and new level of energy in the body. The sounds balance the five zones of the left and right hemispheres of the brain to activate the Neutral Mind or Shuniya.

RA (sun) **MA** (moon) **DA** (earth) **SA** (impersonal Infinity ascending and expanding)
SA (impersonal Infinity descending as ether mingling with earth)
SAY (personal feeling of sacred *Thou* or embodiment of Sa)
SO (personal sense of merger)
HUNG (Infinite vibrating and real) (So Hung = *I am Thou.*)

1. Sit in Easy Pose with a light Jalandhar bandh.

2. Have the elbows tucked comfortably against the ribs. Extend the forearms out at a 45 degree angle out from the center of the body. The palms are flat, facing up, the wrists pulled back, fingers together, and thumbs spread. Consciously keep the palms flat during the meditation. The Mantra consists of eight basic sounds: RA MA DA SA SA SAY SO HUNG

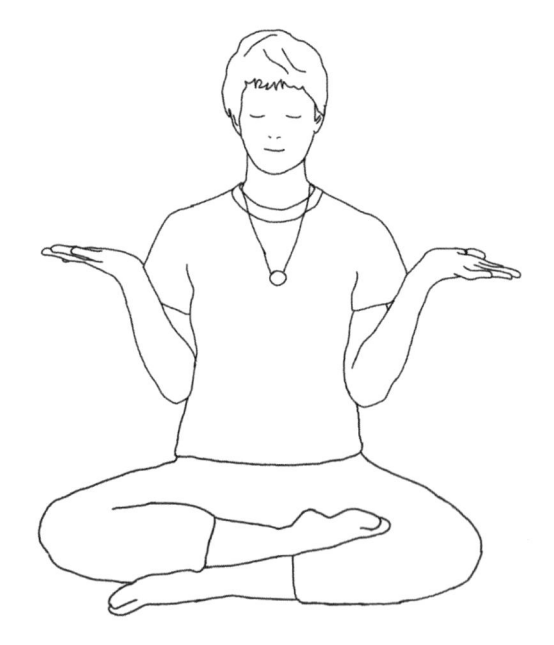

Pull the navel point powerfully on *SO* and *HUNG*. Note that *HUNG* is not long and drawn out. Clip it off forcefully as you pull in the navel. Chant one complete cycle of the entire mantra and then inhale deeply and repeat. To chant this mantra properly, remember to move your mouth fully with each sound. Feel the resonance in your mouth and the sinus areas. Let your mind concentrate on the qualities that are evoked by the combination of sounds.

3. Chant powerfully for 11-31 minutes.

4. To end, inhale deeply and hold the breath as you offer a healing prayer, visualizing the person you wish to heal (including yourself) as being totally healthy, radiant and strong. Imagine the person completely engulfed in healing white light, completely healed. Then exhale and inhale deeply again, hold your breath and offer your prayer. Then, lift your arms up high and vigorously shake out your hands and fingers.

Author's note: To listen to the proper rhythm and sound, go to www.kriteachings.org

tantric meditation

We are designed to face the challenge of tomorrow. To use that potential we must live in the present moment and accept what that moment brings. If we become angry, resentful, or dive into fantasy we lose synchrony with the moment and cannot make an appropriate response.[41]

– Gurucharan Singh Khalsa, Ph. D

Healing Ring of Tantra

When people meditate together, the power of their numbers geometrically multiplies so that the prayer power is squared. With 11 people, you have the meditative prayer power of 121 people (11 x 11). If 20 people meditate together, the prayer power equals 400 people (20 x 20). Everyone's auras are merged in the experience and the prayers of each person are supported and enhanced by the focusing power of the whole group.

The Healing Ring of Tantra meditation engages the individual voice of every participant and the group voice. This ring is a special form of prayer and can be used to generate and direct tremendous healing energy. It is advisable for participants to cover the crown of the head to stay grounded and avoid headaches.

The ring of participants will chant to direct healing energy towards any person: a member of the circle, someone long distance or someone located in the center of the circle. The chant is a call and response form. During the meditation, the ring must never be broken for any reason.

Checkpoints: This meditation in either format is only to be done on a Full Moon, New Moon and 11th day of the New Moon, with a minimum of 11 people.

1. Eleven or more people sit in a comfortable cross-legged position and form an unbroken circle by holding hands.

Author's note: When teaching, I instruct students who need to sit in a chair to make sure they are in the circle and in contact with each person on both sides.

2. Eyes are closed.

3. The mantra goes around the circle, with each person taking a turn to powerfully call out the mantra in monotone, answered by all the members of the circle: WHA-HAY GUROO.

    WHA and HAY each have one beat and GUROO has two beats. The caller then says *SAT NAM* softly, and the person sitting to the left of the caller becomes the next caller. The chant continues in a clockwise direction around the circle. Maintain a constant rhythm.

    Inhale as the mantra is being chanted by the caller; exhale as you chant the mantra in response. The participants should focus their minds to listen and let themselves be filled with the sound, acutely tuning into the call and then answering.

4. Continue for 11 and not longer than 31 minutes.

Spiral Format

Another way to do this meditation is with the participants seated to create a spiral. They join hands, alternately facing in opposite directions. (The left hand of one person will hold the right hand of the person to their right.) If there are people of both genders, the seating in the spiral should alternate between male and female. Same gender individuals can complete the outer tail of the spiral. The person seated in the center of the spiral, if possible, should be a woman. The person seated in the center and the one in the outermost position of the spiral should hold the palms of each of their free hands facing up, to connect with the infinite.

The chanting begins with the person seated in the center and proceeds to the next person in the spiral until the outermost person chants. Then the chanting proceeds back to the center person.

journaling after yoga [41A]

To serve body, mind and spirit, a comprehensive Yoga practice includes self-reflection. Your Yoga practice is opening your awareness to more expansive states of peace and self-discovery. There is no better time for journaling, which can also include drawing and poetry. If you feel some resistance to this idea, just have a pen and paper ready when you finish your practice. Writing from present moment awareness is a powerful practice. See what happens.

Yogi Bhajan often asked his students to write on a given topic to analyze themselves in a self-reflective manner or journal experiences past or present. This kind of journaling is different from simply doing a diary or a descriptive summary of events or personal feelings. These can be done without self-reflection, without a shift in perspective and without assessing how you could apply the techniques and skills to actual situations. This process is a learning journal and it will increase your capacity to step back from the flow of thoughts and feelings to establish a perspective on yourself through consciousness.

To journal in this way, you will record observations about yourself, the world, your experiences, and your practice. Reflecting on that from multiple perspectives will strengthen the habit to process your life with intuitive insight and critical assessment. This is care for your Self.

You can choose to use the basics: paper and a writing instrument. Or use a computer. Or use an artist's journal. Pick what is comfortable for you. To watch the unfolding of your efforts, it takes some time, patience, consistency, and discipline. Journal every day for at least 40 days and 120 days is recommended in order to watch the unfolding of your efforts and make the skills you acquire conscious and seamlessly sewn into your life.

Journal Format

For each day you write in five ways:

1. Take a few deep breaths. Become still. Open yourself to everything you felt, observed, imagined, and did this day. Become open without censorship or editing. Begin to write. You may flow in your writing. You may jump from experience to idea to feeling –as you wish. It is your unique expression. For example, you might note how you spoke with friends, enemies and colleagues; how a critical news event involved good or poor communication; what insight you received from reading a familiar scripture or inspirational source; or how you became unconscious in an interaction and how you would do it differently in the future. Write as long as you like.

2. Look over what you just wrote. Now, from the perspective of the negative mind, write about the same things. The negative mind filters experiences to protect you, to recognize what is wrong and alert you to error.

3. Immediately write about the same experiences from the perspective of the positive mind. The positive mind filters experiences to find opportunity, things you want, ways to expand or move forward, and skills, feelings or actions you want to use or improve.

4. Get into your neutral mind. Now, look at both of these perspectives, the negative and positive minds. The neutral mind assesses everything from the perspective of your consciousness, identity, intuition, and short and long-term consequences. Write quickly about what you note from this perspective- insights, implications, values demonstrated, integrity in your actions, and recognition of positive and negative effects.

5. Go beyond thought for a moment. Enter into the state of zero (*shuniya*) and from You within you, write a comment. It is a comment between you and yourself, simple, direct and real. It need not be profound or clever, just real within you. It is often short.

Once you try this process a few times, it begins to be easy and flows as you turn the facets of each part of your mind and consciousness to reflect on what you have observed, experienced and done.

Some years ago when visiting China, I came upon a stupa on a mountaintop near Guilin. It had writing embossed in gold on it, and I asked my Chinese host what it meant. 'It means Buddha,' he said. 'Why are there two characters rather than one?' I asked. 'One,' he explained, 'means man. The other means no. And the two together means Buddha.' I stood there in awe. The character for Buddha already contained the whole teaching of the Buddha, and for those who have eyes to see, the secret of life. Here are the two dimensions that make up reality, thingness and no-thingness, form and denial of form, which is the recognition that form is not who you are.[42]

— Eckhart Tolle

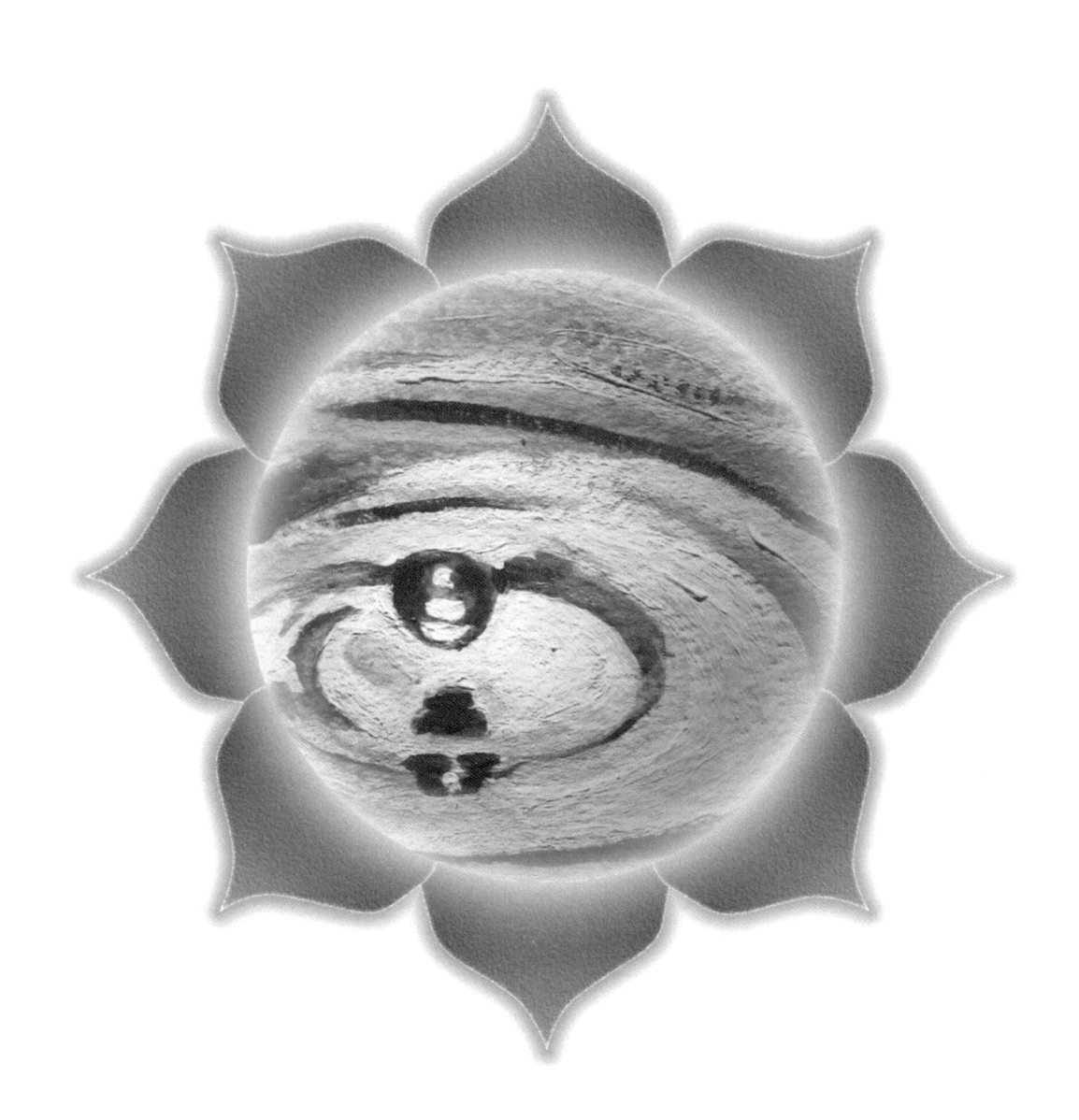

source glossary

The Shambala Encyclopedia of Yoga, Georg Feuerstein, Ph.D

The Yoga Tradition, Georg Feuerstein, Ph.D

The Master's Touch, Yogi Bhajan, Ph.D

Kundalini Yoga: The Flow of Eternal Power, Shakti Parwha Kaur Khalsa

Kundalini Yoga: As Taught By Yogi Bhajan, Shakta Kaur Khalsa

The Teachings of Ramana Maharshi, edited by David Godman

Reaching Me In Me, compiled and illustrated by Harijot Kaur Kalsa, Kundalini Research Institute

Self Knowledge, compiled and illustrated by Harijot Kaur Kalsa, Kundalini Research Institute

Praana Praanee Praanayam, compiled and illustrated by Harijot Kaur Kalsa, Kundalini Research Institute

The Sacred Circle Tarot, Anna Franklin and Illustrated by Paul Mason

The Aquarian Teacher Yoga Manual, Kundalini Research Institute

Divine Alignment, Guru Prem Singh Khalsa and Harijot Kaur Khalsa

One Taste, Ken Wilber

Integral Life Practice, Ken Wilber, Terry Patten, Adam Leonard, Marco Morelli, Integral Books

Integral Spirituality, Ken Wilber

A Thousand Names For Joy, Byron Katie

A New Earth, Eckhart Tolle

The Power of Now, Eckhart Tolle

The Synthesis of Yoga, Sri Aurobindo

To order a CD of musical notations for the Chanting Meditations please contact the author at www.oneheartfourseasons.com.

glossary of gurmuki and sanskrit terms

Adi Mantra | *Adi* means primal or first and *mantra* means to think. Usually expressed as sounds or syllables or words to invoke the infinite mind.

Ajna | Command Wheel. Third-Eye or Sixth Chakra located between the eyebrows and associated with the pituitaty gland.

Amrit Vela | Ambrosial time, 2 1/2 hours before the sun rises.

Anahata | Wheel of the unstruck sound, located at the heart center.

Asana | Seat or posture.

Ashram | A hermitage where disciples exert themselves in a sacred way of life.

Aura | An energy center. The electromagnetic field which surrounds every living creature, the Eighth Chakra.

Bandha, Bandhas | Bond or bondage, lock or constriction that stops the flow of prana within the body.

Bhaja Man Mere Hari Ka Nam Sat Nam | My mind dwells in the true identity of the infinite.

Bhujangasana | Cobra Pose.

Buddhi Mind | Feminine form of Buddha consciousness.

Citta | Mind or consciousness, enlightened mind.

Chakras | Wheel of movement, energy centers of consciousness associated with seven nerve centers in the body and the aura.

Drishti | View, gaze, focal point.

Gurmuki | From the Guru's mouth, a phonetic dialect off Sanskrit.

Guru | *Gu* means darkness, *ru* means light. That which takes ones consciousness form darkness to light.

Gyan Mudra | Hand gesture to seal the intellect.

Har | The infinite connected to prosperity and the green energy of money.

Hatha Yoga | Forceful Yoga, self-realization by means of perfecting the physical body.

Jalandhar Bandh | Contraction of the throat, throat lock practiced in conjunction with postures and mudras.

Karnee | creativity.

Kriya | Complete act.

Kundalini | Serpent power, A psycho-spiritual force.

Manipura | Third Chakra located at the navel.

Glossary of Gurmuki and Sanskrit Terms (continued)

Mantra | To think, usually expressed as sounds or syllables or words to invoke the infinite mind.

Mula bandh | Root Lock, one of the three body. locks, to contract the perineum and draw the navel toward the spinal column.

Muladhara | Root-prop wheel, the First Chakra located at the perineum or anus, pertains to the earth element.

Naad | Sound.

Prana | Life, breathing forth.

Pranayam | Breath control.

Raj Yoga | Royal Yoga, Classical Yoga.

Rajas, Rajasic | Affected, excited.

Sadhana | Daily practice as a means of realization.

Sahasrara | Crown Chakra, the top-most center of the body's psycho-spiritual energy.

Sanskrit | Ancient language originating in India.

Sat Nam | True name or true identity.

Sattva, Sattvic, Beingness | Immaculate, illuminating without ill.

Shakti | Power, feminine, Divine consort of Shiva.

Shiva | Benevolent, masculine form of the Divine.

Shuniya | A state or stage of consciousness where the ego is dissolved into a state of *zero*.

Sitali | Making the sound, breath control.

Sri Aurobindo | Indian philosopher, political activist, mystic, and spiritual leader of the 20th century.

Standing Straight | Samasthiti.

Subagh | Fortunate.

Surya Namaskara | Sun Salutation.

Svadisthana Own | base center, the Second Chakra located at the genitals, associated with water.

Tamas, Tamasic | Darkness, inertia, heedlessness, sleep, sloth.

Tantra | Loom, to extend, to expand, instructions to activate the Kundalini power.

Tao | *Tao Te Ching*: Chinese classic spiritual book about enlightenment.

Tapas | internal heat.

Uddiyana Bandh | Upward lock, great lock, which uses all three body locks: diaphragm, neck and root.

glossary of gurmuki and sanskrit terms (continued)

Vishudda | Pure wheel, the Fifth Chakra located at the throat.

Yogi Bhajan | Harbhajan Singh Khalsa, (1929-2004), Kundalini Yoga master, emigrated to the US in 1968, created Healthy Happy Holy Organization (3HO) to bring Kundalini Yoga and Sikhism to the West.

Yogi Ramana Maharshi | One of the significant spiritual teachers to emerge from India in the early 1900s.

Wahe Guru | Wow! The Wisdom! Indescribable is the ecstasy of the wisdom that brings us from darkness to Light!

bibliography

Allione Tsultrim.
Women of Wisdom.
Ithaca, NY: Snow Lion Pub., 2000

Bhajan, Yogi, Ph.D.
The Master's Touch: On Being a Sacred Teacher For the New Age.
Espanola, NM: Kundalini Resaearch Institute, 2000.

Feuerstein, Georg.
The Shambala Encyclopedia of Yoga.
Boston: Shambala Pub. Inc., 1997.

Feuerstein, Georg.
The Yoga Tradition: It's History, Literature, Philosophy and Practice.
Prescott AZ: Hohm Press, 2001.

Franklin, Anna.
The Sacred Circle Tarot: A Celtic Pagan Journey.
Woodbury, MN:Llewylln, 2006.

Godman, David, editor.
Be As You Are: The Teachings of Sri Ramana Maharshi.
New York: Penguin, 1992.

Judith, Anodea.
Wheels of Life; A User's Guide to the Chakra System.
St Paul, MN: Llewllyn, 1994.

Judith, Anodea and Selene Vega.
The Sevenfold Journey: Reclaiming Mind, Body, & Spirit Through the Chakras.
U.S.A.: Judith & Vega,1993.

Katie, Byron.
A Thousand Names For Joy: Living in Harmony with the Way Things Are.
New York: Harmony Books, 2007.

Khalsa, Dharma Singh, Ph.D., and Cameron Stauth.
Meditation as Medicine: Activate the Power of Your Natural Healing Force.
New York: Fireside, 2002.

Khalsa, Gurucharan Sing, Ph.D., compiled.
Kundalini Yoga: Guidelines For Sadhana (Daily Practice).
Espanola NM: Kundalini Research Institute, 1999.

Khalsa, Guru Dharam Singh and Darryl O'Keefe.
The Kundalini Yoga Experience; Bringing Body, Mind, and Spirit Together.
New York: Fireside, 2002.

Khalsa, Harijot Kaur, complied and illustrated. *Reaching Me In Me: Kundalini Yoga As Taught By Yogi Bhajan.*
Espanola, NM: Kundalini Research Institute, 2002.

Khalsa, Harijot Kaur, complied and illustrated.
Self Experience: Kundalini Yoga As Taught By Yogi Bhajan.
Espanola, NM: Kundalini Research Institute, 2000.

Khalsa, Harijot Kaur, complied and illustrated.
Physical Wisdom: Kundalini Yoga As Taught By Yogi Bhajan.
Espanola, NM: Kundalini Research Institute, 2001.

Khalsa, Guru Prem Singh.
Divine Alignment.
Espanola, NM: Guru prem Singh Khalsa and Harijot Kaur Khalsa, 2003.

bibliography (continued)

Khalsa, Sat Kripal Kaur, Ph.D., consulting editor.
Kundalini Yoga For Youth & Joy.
Espanola, NM: YB Teachings, 1983.

Khalsa, Shakta Kaur.
Kundalini Yoga: Unlock Your Inner Potential Through Life-Changing Exercise.
New York: Dorling Kindersley, 2001.

Khalsa, Shakta Kaur.
Yoga for Women: Health and Radiant beauty for Every Stage Of life.
New York: Dorling Kindersley, 2002.

Khalsa, Shakti Parwha Kaur.
Kundalini Postures and Poetry: An Illustrated Handbook of Classic Yoga Poses as taught By the Master Yogi Bhajan, Ph.D.
New York:Perigee, 2003.

Swami Muktananda
Play of Consciousness
South Fallsburg NY: Syda Foundation, 1978.

Schiffmann, Erich.
Yoga: The Spirit and Practice of Moving Into Stillness.
New York: Pocket Books, 1996.

Sri Aurobindo
The Integral Yoga: Sri Aurobindo's Teachng and Method of Practice.
Twin Lakes WI: Lotus Press, 1993

Sri Aurobindo
The Synthesis of Yoga.
Twin Lakes WI: Lotus Press,1996

Sri Aurobindo
The Divine Life
Twin Lakes Wi: Lotus Press, 2006

Thompson, George
The Bhagavad Gita: A New Translation
New York: North Point Press, 2008.

Tolle, Eckhart.
The Power Of Now: A Guide to Spiritual Enlightenment.
Novato CA: New World Library, 1999 and
Vancouver B.C. Canada: Namaste Publishing, 1999.

Tolle, Eckhart.
A New Earth: Awakening to Your Life's Purpose.
New York: Penguin, 2005.

Wilber, Ken.
One Taste: Daily Reflections on Integral Spirituality.
Boston: Shambala Pub. Inc., 2000.

Wilber, Ken.
Integral Vision: A Very Short Introduction to the Revolutionary Integral Approach to Life, God, the Universe, and Everything.
Boston: Shambala Pub. Inc., 2007.

Wilber, Ken.
Integral Spirituality: A Startling New Role for Religion in the Modern and Postmodern World.
Boston: Integral Books, 2006.

references

Preface

1. Yogi Bhajan: *The Yoga Tradition*, page 336-337, George Feuerstein (Hohm Press 2001)

Using This Book

1A. Sanskrit: Wikipedia definition.
1B. Gurmukhi: Wikipedia definition.
2. Sat Nam: *Kundalini Yoga: As Taught By Yogi Bhajan*, page 16, Shakta Kaur Khalsa (Dorling Kindersley 2001)
3. Sat means Being: *The Shambala Encyclopedia of Yoga*, page 263, George Feuerstein (Shambala Pub. Inc. 1997)
3A. Yogi Bhajan quote: *The Master's Touch*, page 94 (Kundalini Research Institute 2000
3B. Yogi Bhajan quote: From Yogi Bhajan lecture entitled "The Self-Sensory System and the Transition of the Piscean Age to the Aquarian Age" August 1, 2000, page 11, (The Self-Sensory Human, Curriculum Guidelines compiled by M.S.S. Guruka Singh Khalsa (IKYTA Teachers Curriculum 2003), Espanola, New Mexico)

Solstice and Equinox

3C. www.3HO.org http://3ho.org/events/WinterSolstice/wintersol.about.html)
4. Ramana Maharshi Quote: *Be As You Are*, The Teachings of Sri Ramana Maharshi, page 16, edited by David Godman (Penguin Books 1992)

My Practice

5. Adi Mantra (Ong Namo Guru Dev Namo): The Aquarian Teacher Yoga Manual, page 54, 78 (Kundalini Research Institute 2003)

Getting Started

6. Prepare for Yoga: *The Aquarian Teacher Yoga Manual*, page 247, (Kundalini Research Institute 2003)
7. More Prepare For Yoga: *The Aquarian Teacher Yoga Manual*, page 135, (Kundalini Research Institute 2003)

Yoga Kriyas

8. Patanjali: *The Aquarian Teacher Yoga Manual*, pages 38-41, (Kundalini Research Institute 2003)
9. Kriya: *The Aquarian Teacher Yoga Manual*, page 100, (Kundalini Research Institute 2003)

Practicing

10. Warm-ups: *The Aquarian Teacher Yoga Manual*, page 102 and 281, (Kundalini Research Institute 2003)
11. Practice Meditation or Kriya for a Specific Time: *Kundalini Yoga: As Taught By Yogi Bhajan*, page 157, Shakta Kaur Khalsa (Dorling Kindersley 2001)

Body Locks to Seal Energy

12. Root Lock or Mulbandh: *Divine Alignment,*

references (continued)

page 4-8, Guru Prem Singh Khalsa, Guru Prem Singh Khalsa and Harijot Kaur Khalsa 2003)

12A. Upanishads quote, Manipura: *The Aquarian Teacher Yoga Manual*, page 180 (Kundalini Research Institute 2003)

13. Neck Lock or Jalandhar Bandh: *Divine Alignment*, page 9-13, Guru Prem Singh Khalsa, Guru Prem Singh Khalsa and Harijot Kaur Khalsa 2003)

14. Diaphragm Lock or Uddiyana Bandh: *Divine Alignment*, page 18-20, Guru Prem Singh Khalsa, Guru Prem Singh Khalsa and Harijot Kaur Khalsa 2003)

14A. Great Lock or Mahabandh: *The Aquarian Teacher Yoga Manual*, page 109, (Kundalini Research Institute 2003)

Breath (Pranayam)

15. Pranayam: *The Aquarian Teacher Yoga Manual*, page 91, (Kundalini Research Institute 2003)

15A. Yogi Bhajan Quote, Pranayam: *The Aquarian Teacher Yoga Manual*, page 89, (Kundalini Research Institute 2003)

16. Breath Frequency: *The Aquarian Teacher Yoga Manual*, page 91 (Kundalini Research Institute 2003)

17. Long Deep Breathing in Three Parts/Prana: *The Shambhala Encyclopedia of Yoga*, page 224, Georg Fereurstein, Shambhala 2000.

18. Breath of Fire: *The Aquarian Teacher Yoga Manual*, page 95, (Kundalini Research Institute 2003)

19. Right and Left Notril Breathing: *The Aquarian Teacher Yoga Manual*, page 96, (Kundalini Research Institute 2003)

20. Sitali Pranayam: *The Aquarian Teacher Yoga Manual*, page 97, (Kundalini Research Institute 2003)

21. One Minute Breath: *The Aquarian Teacher Yoga Manual*, page 91, (Kundalini Research Institute 2003)

22. Suspending the Breath: *The Aquarian Teacher Yoga Manual*, page 93, (Kundalini Research Institute 2003)

Mantra

23. Chanting: *The Aquarian Teacher Yoga Manual*, page 66, (Kundalini Research Institute 2003)

24. Naad: *The Aquarian Teacher Yoga Manual*, page 67, (Kundalini Research Institute 2003)

Mudra / Hand Positions

25. Mudra: *The Aquarian Teacher Yoga Manual*, page 105-106, (Kundalini Research Institute 2003)

Focal Point for Your Eyes

26. Focal Point: The Aquarian Teacher Yoga Manual, page 136, (Kundalini Research Institute 2003)

27. Byron Katie Quote: A Thousand names For Joy, page 125, Byron Katie, (Harmony Books 2007)

Meditation

28. Mind: *The Aquarian Teacher Yoga Manual*, page 120-121, (Kundalini Research Institute 2003)

references (continued)

How to Sit, Stand and Bend

28A. Compression and Tension: the DVD, *Anatomy of Yoga*, by Paul Grilley. Find him at www.paulgrilley.com.

29. Seated Poses: *The Aquarian Teacher Yoga Manual*, page 103-104, (Kundalini Research Institute 2003)

30. Ken Wilber Quote: One Taste: *Daily Reflections on Integral Spirituality*, page 276, (Shambhala 2000)

Energy Centers in the Body/ Chakras

31. Chakras: *The Aquarian Teacher Yoga Manual*, pages 183-195, (Kundalini Research Institute 2003)

32. Yogi Bhajan Quote: *Reaching Me In Me*, page 9, compiled and illustrated by Harijot Kaur Khalsa, (Kundalini Research Institute 2002)

33. Ken Wilber's Integral Map Of Consciousness: *Integral Life Practice*, page 90-98, Ken Wilber, Terry Patten, Adam Leonard, Marco Morelli (Integral Books 2008)

33A. Ken Wilber Quote: *Integral Spirituality* pages 258-259 (Shambhala Publications) 2007

Ten Bodies

34. Ten Bodies: The Aquarian Teacher Yoga Manual, page 200-204, (Kundalini Research Institute 2003)

Tune in to Begin

34A. Gurucharan Singh Khalsa Ph.D quote: *Self Knowledge*, page 4, compiled and illustrated by Harijot Kaur Khalsa, (Kundalini Research Institute 2001)

35. Adi Mantra: *The Aquarian Teacher Yoga Manual*, page 54, (Kundalini Research Institute 2003)

36. Complete Adi Mantra For Individual Meditation: *The Aquarian Teacher Yoga Manual*, page 413, (Kundalini Research Institute 2003)

Practice for Present Moment Awareness

37. With each exercise and kriya: : *Reaching Me In Me*, page IV-V, compiled and illustrated by Harijot Kaur Khalsa, (Kundalini Research Institute 2002)

To End

38. Longtime Sunshine and Sat Nam to end: *The Aquarian Teacher Yoga Manual*, page 283, (Kundalini Research Institute 2003)

Always

39. Sri Aurobindo Quote: *The Synthesis of Yoga*, un-numbered page before the Introduction (Lotus Press 1996)

39A. Sri Aurobindo Quote: *The Synthesis of Yoga*, page 7 (Lotus Press 1996)

A Meditation and Kriya For All Seasons

40. Yogi Bhajan Quote: *Self Experience*, page VII, compiled and illustrated by Harijot Kaur Khalsa, (Kundalini Research Institute 2000)

references (continued)

Tantric Ring

41. Gurucharan Singh Khalsa Ph.D quote: *Self Knowledge*, page 44, compiled and illustrated by Harijot Kaur Khalsa, (Kundalini Research Institute 2001)

Journaling After Yoga

41A. Journaling: *KRI Internaltional Teacher Training Level 2: Vitality and Stress Study Guide*, pages 79-81, (Kundalini Research Institute 2008)

42. Eckhart Tolle Quote: *A New Earth*, page 221, Eckhart Tolle (Dutton 2005)

A Meditation and Kriya for All Seasons

Beginner's Meditation: *Kundalini Yoga*, page 158, Shakta Kaur Khalsa (Dorling Kindersley 2001)
Sat Kriya: *The Aquarian Teacher Yoga Manual*, page 348, (Kundalini Research Institute 2003)

Spring Equinox

Energizing Series: *Kundalini Yoga: As Taught By Yogi Bhajan*, page 46-47, Shakta Kaur Khalsa (Dorling Kindersley 2001)
Energizing Series: *The Aquarian Teacher Yoga Manual*, page 321 (stretch pose), (Kundalini Research Institute 2003)

Hip Stretches

Butterfly & Butterfly Bend: *The Aquarian Teacher Yoga Manual*, page 312, (Kundalini Research Institute 2003)
Triangle: *The Aquarian Teacher Yoga Manual*, page 321, (Kundalini Research Institute 2003)
Basic Spinal Energizer Series: *The Aquarian Teacher Yoga Manual*, page 339, (Kundalini Research Institute 2003)
Wahe Guru Kriya: *The Aquarian Teacher Yoga Manual*, page 380, (Kundalini Research Institute 2003) and Kundalini Yoga: As Taught By Yogi Bhajan, page 98, Shakta Kaur Khalsa (Dorling Kindersley 2001)
Fight Brain Fatigue: *Self Experience*, page 35, compiled by Harijot Kaur Khalsa (Kundalini Research Institute 2000)
The Divine Shield Meditation For Protection and Positivity: *The Aquarian Teacher Pilot Manual*, page 429, (Kundalini Research Institute 2002-03)

Midsummer Solstice

Sun Salutations: *Divine Alignment*, pages 54-59, (Guru Prem Singh Khalsa 2003)
Abdominal Strengthening: *Kundalini Yoga: Guidelines For Sadhana*, page 57-58, (Kundalini Research Institute 1996)
Strengthening the Aura: *Kundalini Yoga: Guidelines For Sadhana*, page 59, (Kundalini Research Institute 1996)
Karnee Kriya: *Praana Praanee Praanayam*, page 89, Compiled From the Teachings of Yogi Bhajan by Harijot Kaur Khalsa (Kundalini Research Institute 2006)

references (continued)

Bhaja Mane Mere: *Angel's Waltz*, CD track 6, Sada Sat Kaur Khalsa. Not KRI Approved.

Autumn Equinox

Spinal Series: : *Kundalini Yoga: As Taught By Yogi Bhajan*, page 48-55, Shakta Kaur Khalsa (Dorling Kindersley 2001)

Life Nerve Stretch (Front Stretch and Left and Right): *The Aquarian Teacher Yoga Manual*, page 316, (Kundalini Research Institute 2003)

Pituitary Gland Series: *The Aquarian Teacher Yoga Manual*, page 373, (Kundalini Research Institute 2003)

Creative Meditation of the Sublime Self: *Reaching Me in Me*, page 47-48, compiled by Harijot Kaur Khalsa, (Kundalini Research Institute 2002)

The Ancient Way of Prayer: *Praana Praanee Praanayam*, page 94-95, compiled by Harijot Kaur Khalsa (Kundalini Research Institute 2006))

Sat Narayan: "The instructions for this meditation are from the contemporaneous notes of Susan Q. Brown and could not be verified by KRI Review."

Midwinter Solstice

Cat-Cow: *The Aquarian Teacher Yoga Manual*, page 313, (Kundalini Research Institute 2003)

Child's (Baby) Pose: *The Aquarian Teacher Yoga Manual*, page 311, (Kundalini Research Institute 2003)

Archer Pose: *The Aquarian Teacher Yoga Manual*, page 311, (Kundalini Research Institute 2003)

Frog Pose: *The Aquarian Teacher Yoga Manual*, page 315, (Kundalini Research Institute 2003)

Self- Adjustment of the Spine: : *Kundalini Yoga: As Taught By Yogi Bhajan*, page 62-63, Shakta Kaur Khalsa (Dorling Kindersley 2001)

Subagh Kriya: *Self Experience*, page 43-44, compiled by Harijot Kaur Khalsa (Kundalini Research Institute 2000)

Burn Inner Anger: *Praana Praanee Praanayam*, page 147, compiled by Harijot Kaur Khalsa (Kundalini Research Institute 2006)

Siri Gaitri Mantra: *The Aquarian Teacher Yoga Manual*, page 422, (Kundalini Research Institute 2003)

Healing Ring of Tantra: *The Aquarian Teacher Yoga Manual*, page 421, (Kundalini Research Institute 2003)

Season Sections / Attributes

Spring Equinox: *The Sacred Circle Tarot*, page 149-151, Anna Franklin and Illustrated by Paul Mason, (Llewellyn Publications 2006)

Midsummer Solstice: *The Sacred Circle Tarot*, page 193-196, Anna Franklin and Illustrated by Paul Mason, (Llewellyn Publications 2006)

Autumn Equinox: *The Sacred Circle Tarot*, page 234-236, Anna Franklin and Illustrated by Paul Mason, (Llewellyn Publications 2006)

Midwinter Solstice: *The Sacred Circle Tarot*, page 282-285, Anna Franklin and Illustrated by Paul Mason, (Llewellyn Publications 2006)

notes

notes

notes